DEAFNESS IN

Looks at different types c
condition affects sufferers, ar
coping with the day-to-day pi
exercises.

DEAFNESS IN THE ADULT

What Hearing Loss Means and What Can Be Done to Help

by

Winifred Brinson

THORSONS PUBLISHING GROUP
Wellingborough * New York

First published 1986

© WINIFRED BRINSON 1986

British Library Cataloguing in Publication Data

Brinson, Winifred
  Deafness in the adult: what a hearing loss means
  and what can be done to help.
  1. Deafness
  I. Brinson, Winifred
  617.8   RF290

  ISBN 0-7225-1251-1

Printed and bound in Great Britain

CONTENTS

FOREWORD

The consequences of deafness are so complex and far reaching as to baffle even those who suffer from it. Those who are born deaf perhaps never quite understand its ramifications and maybe never really miss what they never knew. For those who become deaf, the catalogue of consequences unfolds slowly, according to the development of deafness, or is exposed dramatically if they are deafened suddenly or totally.

When hearing fades some adjustment is necessary to a different but still basically familiar world. Communication is still aural, but supplemented by a hearing aid and some lipreading. But for those who are totally deafened, major adjustment is required. Communication depends entirely on sight as all the normal hearing clues have vanished.

The loss of environmental sounds is the most obvious. The daily roar of traffic, the useful ringing of a telephone or door bell and the glories of music are strikingly absent. Yet the fundamental loss to a totally deaf person is the human voice. The inability to understand others leads to tension, frustration, misunderstanding and, worst of all, isolation.

Added to all this, when deafness is total, is its effect on the deaf person's voice. In the absence of any feedback it is impossible to monitor speech, so the pitch, modulation, rhythm and level all suffer. There is nothing more noticeable than a 'deaf person's voice'.

This is the bleak, and sometimes tragic, reality of severe or total deafness. It seems devoid of all hope, especially as medical science is in its infancy so far as the treatment of nerve deafness is concerned. But there is hope. More than that, the worst consequences of deafness can be overcome.

Not all of the problems can be solved by any means. Yet by acquiring some skill in lipreading, and by using the benefits of speech therapy, a deaf person can come to terms with deafness and, if the will is there, live a happy and fulfilled life.

A great deal depends upon the family, and to some extent friends. Their understanding and co-operation are treasures beyond price for the deaf person. Among the public some will understand and be willing to help, while others are either indifferent or cannot comprehend deafness and find it easier to turn away. However, most people willingly co-operate, especially if the deaf person has acquired some skill in lipreading and is able to speak reasonably clearly.

Generally speaking, public attitudes toward deaf people have improved very considerably in recent years. To some extent deafness can even be turned to advantage for people become interested when they see a deaf person using lip-reading skills.

While an emotional reaction to deafness is understandable tackling it in a practical fashion, by learning lipreading, makes it less of a catastrophe.

This means hard work, constant practice, intense concentration and skilled professional advice.

Winifred Brinson has devoted her life to teaching deaf people the arts of lipreading and clear speech. She has a profound understanding of their problems and a deep insight into the complexities of deafness. Her keen sensitivity and deep knowledge make her one of the finest teachers I have ever known.

Her book has something for those with all kinds of deafness. She recognises very clearly the difficulties facing deaf people and displays an encyclopaedic knowledge of the answers. In this book she has made a valuable contribution toward a better life for deaf people.

The Rt Hon Jack Ashley CH MP

INTRODUCTION

'There's none so deaf as those that won't hear,' (old proverb), or *'she hears when she wants to'*. Perhaps this proverb arose from ignorance of the true problems relating to deafness in adult life. Certainly, and thankfully, only a small proportion of adults suffer a total loss of hearing; but for those with partial hearing there are many misconceptions in the public mind that have to be faced, apart from coming to terms with the handicap. Deafness, like the word blindness, is a blanket term. But, unlike the latter, it is far more difficult to imagine a life lived without hearing than it is to imagine oneself unable to see. The horror of losing light and colour and space in adult life is indeed frightening, but it is also true to say that deafness can be even more frightening if we have the understanding and imagination to know what it would mean. It is a far more complicated matter than just not being able to hear sound and, in this book, I hope to make clear just what a hearing loss means, not only to the sufferer but to his immediate family, friends and social circle.

There are many excellent technical books on the performance and use of hearing aids; books abound on the physics of sound and the science of audiometry; there are fewer but still useful books on the subject of lipreading; and there is a growing literature on the need for all-round rehabilitation for the deafened adult. But this book seeks to touch on all these in a practical, non-technical manner related to my own experience of work with the deaf over the past forty years.

We can glibly say of a person, 'Oh he's deaf'. But are we talking about a child born with such a severe loss that he

can never know the concept of sound as we know it? Are
we speaking of a child with partial hearing at birth, or one
who acquires a loss, perhaps from measles or an attack of
meningitis, after he has learned to speak? Are we speaking
of a young adult with one damaged ear-drum, or one who
has a high-frequency loss in both ears? Are we speaking of
an older person who has slowly become more and more
deaf over a long period of time? Are we speaking of an adult
who is able to make use of a hearing aid? Or are we speaking
of someone who has suffered a traumatic deafness that cut
off all meaningful sounds for them overnight? There are
many categories of deafness.

I shall not be including the problems of deafness in
childhood in this book, since recognition of the child's
needs and facilities for special education have long been in
operation. However, this is not the case in respect of the
deafened adult so, although I may need to speak of some of
the early problems of hearing loss, I shall endeavour to
describe what it means to be deafened in any way in adult
life, although differing degrees of deafness will require
varying degrees of understanding and advice.

What the blind person does not lose with his sight is the
ability to communicate — in fact, if a blind man sat in a
darkened room with a sighted friend nothing would hinder
their normal flow of speech and conversation. And despite
word processors, telex machines, typewriters, and visual
communicators such as Ceefax, Prestel and Teletext, we
still rely on talking to people, however unimportant the
subject matter might be, to maintain our warm, social
relationships and to feel a part of the community. Deafness
does not allow this. Even a slight loss, particularly one
which involves the higher tones of speech, will result in a
lack of precision, which can easily lead to misunderstandings and feelings of tension. This problem becomes
compounded with an ever-increasing hearing loss, and the
adult who has the misfortune to lose all hearing literally
overnight will have enormous, sometimes insurmountable,
difficulties to face. Not only does this apply to the sufferer,
but a spouse will also find his or her life utterly changed and
the ripples of change flow out to affect the whole family.

I am not trying to prove that deafness is a deadly
handicap — on the contrary people are losing their hearing

every day and it is said that we start to lose our hearing as soon as we are born — and, since the span of life increases each century, the numbers of deafened adults will also increase. But I am trying to show that deafness is the least understood of handicaps and that much could be done to alleviate the problems of deaf people.

Of course people go on living with their deafness; for some it may be little more than an irritant and may not make too much impact on their daily life, but for the majority it will mean facing up to a loss of ease in communication that means a loss of the normality of life.

Throughout this book, to eliminate irritating repetition, I shall use the pronoun 'he' to indicate the deafened adult, although it is probable that numerically there are far more women with a hearing loss, since women are outliving their spouses by several years. It is also a fact that more women attend classes for lipreading practice but, since it has been shown that women form the greatest number of students overall at *all* further education courses, this may well be the factor involved in lipreading attendance.

PART ONE

1

THE LOSS OF COMMUNICATION

He put this engine to our ears, which made an incessant noise like that of a watermill.
(Gulliver's Travels)

To understand the effects of an acquired hearing loss it is first necessary to think about the functions of the ear and what we mean by the miracle of 'hearing'.

Recently the anatomy of the ear has undergone a great revival, with experiments in cochlea implants and the stimulation of nerve endings within the inner ear. Surgery is obviously going to be the answer to the conquering of deafness, but as it is still in its initial stages it is not likely to benefit many deaf people for many years yet. However, even early results are showing that when just two low sounds are implanted, a great improvement is found in the lipreading skill of the deaf adult and a better monitoring of his own speech. This is to say that we require a feedback of our own voice to maintain our speech pattern and to hear some sounds, however gross, enables us to decipher the rhythmic patterns of spoken language.

This is the first time I have used that word and yet, contrary to all talk of lipreading and auditory training, any rehabilitation programme for the deaf adult must be based on our use of language. If he is to maintain some degree of normal communication then he is forced to do so with the aid of a lipreading skill — in other words to learn a series of clues in order to make sense of the language being used.

Types of Deafness
Hearing consists of picking up tiny disturbances in the air

that are passed through the various mechanisms of the ear to the aural nerve, and hence to the brain, where they will be interpreted. The ear has to convert the outside stimulus into various patterns, to convey information about the loudness of the sound, the harmony, the frequency and the direction from which it came. The three sections of the ear which accomplish this may all malfunction and cause different types of deafness.

People may suffer from a perceptual or nerve deafness, as they are told on their visit to a hospital or hearing aid clinic. Such terms mean little to anyone outside the audiology professions and I have had many clients who, on being asked what they think it means, assure me that they are suffering from their 'nerves'. Unless they are fortunate enough to be able to visit a hearing therapist — and as yet their numbers are in no more than double figures throughout the country — then there is unlikely to be any professional with the time or ability to give a clear, meaningful explanation of what this may mean to the sufferer in everyday life.

Similarly, with the less common form of deafness, low-frequency loss, an explanation is necessary so that the loser is aware of what he will miss through the hearing channels.

It is possible to have both a high and low-frequency loss together, and also added factors such as tinnitus (noises in the head) and poor balance.

Communication

But let us first return to our language and see how losses affect our communication. We all know that sound is energy — a high sound might even break glass, and too much sound might burst our ear-drums. Even to repeat one sound such as 'p' will flutter a piece of paper. Each sound will vary in pitch because of its frequency and since there are few pure sounds in English, many of our letters are a combination of sounds and contain more than one frequency, which an added complication in a hearing loss. Because of this factor it is difficult to make a hearing aid tailored to each person's requirements. If we have an eyesight problem we expect this to be corrected by having lenses made especially for our particular loss of sight, but it is much more difficult to do this for individual hearing losses. (More on this when I consider the use of a hearing aid.)

We know that we have an alphabet of twenty-six letters and could name them in order very quickly — rarely do we think of the sound that each letter makes in a word when we speak. In other words, we may call a letter f (ef) but must remember that it makes the sound fa in a word — father not efather. If we listen when we make that single letter fa we note that it is a very quiet sound — try contrasting it with one of our vowel sounds, such as 'oo', and the difference in volume is considerable.

Many of our consonants have this high, quiet sound and are the first to be lost when hearing fails, which will mean that we are receiving only parts of whatever conversation may be going on and, worse still, we are losing the truly important parts.

Let us take one sentence: — That fisherman has caught five large fish. If we remove the consonants from the sentence we are left with all vowels: a, i, er, a, a, or, i-e, ar, i.

Even in the written form it makes no sense and if spoken, even less. Unfortunately for the deaf, it is the consonants in our language which make it intelligible. Therefore, if we have a high-frequency deafness we *can* still hear but what we hear is rubbish and will leave a deaf person frustrated, irritated and tense, trying to decipher conversation. It is possible that someone will use a sentence which is so familiar and contains so many vowels that we will immediately be able to understand it. 'Ow ar oo?' said in its correct rhythm will be immediately understood — hence the oft-repeated remark 'Oh he hears when he wants to!'

Should we have a low-frequency loss, then we are better off in that we can still receive the sounds that matter but if we hear only f-t clearly, it might be fat or fit or phut and we need to get, and be sure of, the rest of the sentence in order to make a sensible guess.

When our hearing is tested, the results are charted in the form of an audiogram. This hearing graph is rarely explained, so that few clients are able to say exactly what it is they *do* hear and why it is that sometimes they appear to understand and sometimes not.

The Effects of Communication Loss

This difficulty in communicating may have far-reaching effects. Taken to its extreme it could result in job loss, loss of promotion, or the holding on to an unsuitable job for fear of not finding another.

It will certainly affect family conversations. The hearing spouse, who is unlikely to have been given a counselling session, will soon realize that she is wasting her breath to try to speak to her partner unless they are face to face. She will stop using the little asides. She will not want to start a long discussion where she will have to break her chain of thought in order to repeat phrases. And I have known instances where husband and wife say only four familiar phrases to each other all day — 'Breakfast's ready', 'Do you want coffee?', 'Dinner time', and 'What do you want for supper?' Most of us love to talk, yet we find it most irritating to have to repeat ourselves and are more likely not to talk to the deaf person, or to say instead, 'Oh, it doesn't matter,' if they fail to understand us. So the deaf person finds his social outlets very much curtailed and his working situation fraught with greater possibilities for making mistakes, and this in turn affects the personality.

Much will depend on the character and make-up, as well as the lifestyle of individuals. One of my clients, a printer by trade, still retained his cheerful, placid manner although he had a severe hearing loss. At work, in a small firm, he found no difficulty in his job; he had never been a person to mix socially, and was content to return home every night and put his feet up. His wife was a similar placid soul, who put all her energies into church work, so that he just let her talk when they were together, knowing that it would be something to do with her Mothers' Union or Flower Rota, and the fact of deafness did not impinge on their lifestyle at all. Others, in different situations, may find their whole lifestyle shattered, but we have to be careful not to blame all sad results on the factor of deafness. The handicap may sometimes just be the excuse for the intended divorce or separation or job loss, rather than the actual reason.

However, in my experience, it is true to say that a hearing loss, however slight, will affect the loser in some degree because of the communication problem. Advice is needed, particularly in the early stages or when a hearing aid is issued, as to the likely effects, and counselling given to prepare the loser for repercussions that might be expected from the public and at home.

It is only in recent years that any research has been undertaken into the disorders of human communication and its effects. One problem has been that there is no register of deaf persons, as there is with the blind. It would be very difficult to keep the fact of blindness secret, yet it is an odd fact that the deafened adult shows no desire to make his handicap obvious or, sometimes, even to acknowledge it. Perhaps this stems back to the ignorance of believing that deafness was allied with loss of mental powers — deaf and daft — but even with the wide publicity that has brought about a tremendous change in public attitudes today, I have found deaf people unwilling to admit their loss. This means that they suffer even more by constant pretence and are, in consequence, often thought stupid when they misconstrue a remark.

I do not believe in some of the old tales which are mentioned in this respect. One familiar story is that of two people meeting, one of whom is deaf.

Hearing person, 'My brother is being buried tomorrow.'

Deaf person, 'Oh how lovely for you.'

The inference here is that 'buried' and 'married' would be similar lipreading shapes and could therefore be misconstrued. This interpretation rather discards all the other factors that need to be noted along with lipreading the shape of words — that is facial expression of the speaker, tone of voice, and manner. I would think that someone talking about a burial would have a very different expression on his face than if he were mentioning a wedding, and that lipreaders should be trained to watch for such additional clues.

This is not to say that our language is not full of anomolies which cause pitfalls for the deafened and that there must be many times when misunderstandings are bound to occur.

Such misconstructions occur over and over again during lipreading classes. Part of the conquering of any handicap is to be shown why and how such mistakes will occur, learn not to take these to heart (after all, hearing people are not free from hearing errors), and to maintain a sense of humour. This is not easy, but the mistakes *are* often amusing and odd. After all, who would think it possible, when a teacher says, 'It distresses me when my daughters argue,' for someone to read this as, 'It distresses me when my corsets are new.' To be shown that these sentences have an almost identical lipreading shape is to feel less foolish, and perhaps even to cultivate an interest in words and the quirks of language. What distresses the deaf person more than any other factor is that of feeling ignored and left out, particularly from family matters.

They find it hurtful to be excluded from news, however trivial, and arrangements which are made over their head. I doubt if this is intentional on the part of the hearing spouse; she is probably trying to save time or embarrassment and make life easier for him. In company, this attitude may even go so far as the deaf person being treated as mentally defective, with two speakers asking, over his head, 'Does he take sugar?' This can build up a bitterness about the handicap which is quite unjustified and is perhaps the reason why so many deaf people appear to be ashamed of their loss.

I am sure that the public attitude to deafness is gradually changing, but more imagination and understanding is required. We know what we can do to help a blind or a physically-handicapped person — a gentle touch, an offer of an arm, the opening of a door, pointing out obstacles; but it is not so obvious how we might help a deaf person out of a communication difficulty. So here are basic simple suggestions for both the deaf and the hearing which cost little effort other than thought.

Suggestions for the Hearing
These suggestions for the hearing will be helpful when speaking with the deaf.

Speak as clearly as you can.   This needs to be qualified as many people, when asked to speak clearly, begin to shout. If the listener is wearing a hearing aid then his position is made far worse in that he now has a far greater volume impinging on his ear-drums, with consequent distortion. It is clarity which is required, not volume.

Neither is an exaggeration of the mouth required. The

movements of speech are fleeting and, if overdone, cause a visual distortion unrecognizable to the reader.

Try to keep gestures to a minimum. It is important to remember that the deafened adult has not resorted to sign language or other manual forms of communication, methods much appreciated by many born with a severe or total loss of hearing. Therefore, any quick movements near the face are a distraction to a person concentrating on facial movements. The hard of hearing appreciate a speaker who keeps still, looks at them while speaking, and does not indulge in hand waving. It is not possible to lipread a roaming figure.

Do have something to write on. It takes several years of hard work and practice to attain a competent lipreading skill and, as we shall see, our language always presents problems, even to the most proficient.

A word written down is often the only clue needed for the reader to make sense of what is being said and is a useful confirmation in the case of times and dates. A teacher would normally check that important points have been correctly understood, but most speakers would not think to do this.

If there is an impasse, try to change the words you have used. It is asking a great deal for members of the public to know which words and phrases are not lipreadable. If a sentence contains too many invisible shapes (an explanation of which will appear later) then any amount of repetition will not help, and both speaker and reader become upset and frustrated. However, our language is so rich in synonyms, and we have so many ways of saying almost the same thing in a different way, that it is usually possible to rephrase a remark. The rephrasing will often include a different set of shapes or a more familiar rhythm that provides more clues.

As an example, think of some of the ways in which we might say, 'I won't be long.' I'll be with you shortly. I'll see you soon. I'll be there in a little while. Wait for me, I'm nearly ready. Just a minute and I'll be with you. I've almost finished, then I'll be with you. And so on. Some of these phrases are more lipreadable than others, yet convey a similar meaning. One common example is the opening remark, 'It's a nice day, isn't it?' which doesn't contain one lipreadable shape; whereas anyone, without any formal tuition, would be able to read 'What a lovely day.'

Make your enunciation clear.   It seems obvious to say that a speaker should not speak with anything in his mouth or mumble or turn away while talking. If he is trying to hold in a cigarette, or a pencil, or clutch a pipe, then his enunciation will be through clenched teeth. In fact it is a normal way of speech for many people. So many 'good speakers' are understood because we can hear their pleasant voices, but a lipreader requires movement to be able to use his skill and gives up in despair when faced with an immobile mouth. It is rather like trying to lipread a ventriloquist when you cannot hear the dummy.

Speak with some animation.   I hesitate to suggest this since it is often interpreted as 'arm waving'. Words are emotive and, as such, should present clues as to mood and subject matter — you would hardly speak about a funeral with a face creased with laughter.

The pitch of the voice also undergoes change, in fact it is the way in which we distinguish between a statement, a question, and an explanation. For example, I would speak these three sentences in quite different tones of voice:

Smith has just scored.
Smith has just scored?
Smith has just scored!

A hearing aid wearer would pick up a tonal variation with practice and a person too deaf to wear an aid would respond to a varying facial pattern. The muscles of our face will move to lift an eyebrow for the question, or we will open our eyes a little wider and enlarge our mouth for the exclamation, and a lipreader relies on such additional clues for meaning.

Of course, some of us are 'deadpan' and could make a garden party sound like a wake, and perhaps women feel or show their emotions more easily than men, but a deaf person would appreciate being able to use his mental ability on other clues than mere lip movement.

The hearing aid factor.   And a final, very important factor to remember is that, because a person is wearing a hearing aid, this does not mean that he is receiving your voice normally. Only if the deaf person has a not-too-severe loss across the entire range of frequencies that we hear, will the aid bring his hearing to near normal. The aid is a crutch, as is lipreading skill, which together enable the deafened adult to maintain a place in society but it can never be a replacement for normal hearing.

Everyone's loss is different; sound is different, often unrecognizable when first heard through the machine, and it is a sad fact that few people are given training both in the limitations and use of their aid. With training, the deaf adult may learn to recognize sounds which are different to those he formerly heard; he may learn to deal with and ignore distortion; he may learn when best to wear the aid and when it would be better to turn it off; he may learn to combine his remembrance of speech and language to make a sensible guess at meaning; but he will always require a good speech pattern from others to enable him to use his aid adequately.

Suggestions for the Deafened

None of the following suggestions is easy to carry out. Some may not be possible because, however hard the deaf work in a situation, the effort has to be two-way for easy communication.

First, acknowledge your hearing impairment. Of course, if you suffer a traumatic deafness, almost overnight, and are left with a total loss of hearing, then you cannot hide the fact. But so many workers do not admit to their loss, thinking, no doubt, that their job would be in jeopardy, when for their colleagues to know might bring some relief and practical help. I have known teachers retire early, journalists give up their work and nurses leave their careers, unable to cope any longer because of a progressive loss, when an acknowledgement at work might have enabled them to transfer their skills to other departments, before colleagues became irritated with the communication difficulties and sympathy was lost.

It is possible to go on for many years without realizing the onset of deafness. It is easy to turn up the volume on the radio or television, mention that people mumble, and be oblivious to the fact that hearing is deteriorating. It has been said that we begin to lose hearing as soon as we are born, but I think the insidious fact is that we accommodate to a gradual loss in the same manner that people with poor sight are able to manage quite well — until there comes a point when both poor hearing and poor sight become severe.

If hearing does deteriorate over a period of time, then it is highly probable that the adult will already have been watching people's faces and unconsciously have picked up a degree of lipreading skill. Very few adults referred to the Deaf Centre in London are absolute beginners in the lipreading sense. In fact, research shows that people without any hearing loss can lipread fairly well as long as they are not asked to do so over a long stretch of time and outside clinical conditions. The adult who *needs* to lipread must concentrate *all* the time and in all situations. The few who may be classed as true beginners are those totally deafened overnight or within a short period of time, or others for whom English is not their native tongue and who, therefore, have a double difficulty.

If you do realize that your hearing is not as acute as it used to be, or you hear your spouse telling others that you don't hear as well as you did, then it is worth the effort to ask for a hearing test to discover just how great the loss might be. There is no shame attached to this; it is no more your fault that you are forced into wearing a hearing aid than it is that you require spectacles or a prosthesis. All are given to alleviate a problem and help to make life easier and relieve strain.

Study the general situation.   I think that deaf people are more prone to tiredness and tension than the hearing, due to the fact that they must always be observing and mentally alert. Lipreading is so dependent on the mental ability to anticipate and quickly make sense of any clues that the deafened adult needs to be constantly studying a situation, watching a speaker, gauging the roles of the people talking, and whatever is being talked about. Whereas the hearing adult can keep his mind on two things at once, making up a mental shopping list while hearing a friend discuss the weather, the deaf adult must keep his concentration on the matter at hand, trying to stay on the wavelength and hoping that the subject will not suddenly be changed without any clue.

It is quite fun, as a hearing person, to try to do this while in a crowd or when travelling. If you cannot hear people, either because of the background noise or because of distance, try to imagine what they might be saying or judge a mood from their expressions and bodily movements. This will give you an idea of what it is possible to learn without actually hearing speech and the type of clues for which the deaf are always watching.

A hearing aid. More will be said on aids to hearing in a later chapter, but the basic point is to make sure that the aid selected is the best possible for your hearing loss. If it does not seem to be working properly then seek professional advice — it might not be the aid but a change in your hearing that is at fault.

Positioning. It will be up to the deaf adult to put himself in the most favourable light. The hard fact is that *you* are the handicapped one and *you* will need to do the work. If you are not facing the light directly but moving so that the speaker must move to let light fall on his face, then you will be better able to lipread. Try not to be in a situation where you are directly under a loudspeaker: let the hearing person sit there, if there is no other choice, then he will have to raise his voice to hear himself and perhaps enunciate more clearly, which will help you.

Try not to give up. As I shall endeavour to show, it is the beginning of a sentence which often contains unlipreadable words or phrases, and the meaningful words might well come towards the end. Usually it is these words which are the gist of the subject matter and, if you have stayed with the person's mouth, then the very last word could give you the information to enable you to make a sensible answer. Mistakes will be made but this is not limited to the deaf, as hearing people also catch the wrong trains or bring home the wrong goods because they have misheard something. Of course it isn't wise to ask for a repetition while the speaker is still talking, since the latter part of the message may enable you to tell the part you missed, but don't be ashamed to ask people to repeat when you don't understand. After all, as a hearing adult, I use phrases such as 'What did you say?' 'What was that?' 'I beg your pardon?' or even just 'Eh?'.

A sense of humour.   If you have one, then try to maintain it. If you attend a lipreading class or club then you will be shown why mistakes occur, and encouraged to laugh at them, and indeed, many are very comical. If you don't contact other deaf adults, then you will probably never know how confusions arise and it is very easy to become despondent after a series of regrettable mistakes.

Deaf adults usually take one of two courses: they either try to monopolize a conversation, often in an attempt to avoid having to lipread; or they give up all efforts to socialize. Most people like to be listened *to* rather than talked *at*, but if you try to understand what the other person is saying, having explained that you may have difficulty because of your hearing loss, then conversation maintains its two-way activity.

Remember also that lipreading is a skill and, like any other, stales with disuse. Keep practising; there will be bad days, depending on your state of mind and health. It is important to keep up with the national news and your own common activities, as well as adding to your vocabulary, and practising 'in' phrases and colloquialisms that speakers use all the time. In this way you will keep mentally alert, which is an essential part of the skill of lipreading.

What Can the Family Do?
To have a deaf member of a family group can be a shattering experience. In a situation where there is evidently strong emotional attachments, I would feel extremely sorry for the hearing members of the family who were at a loss as how best to help the deaf member or parent.

Spontaneous speech is the least laborious and much the quickest means of communicating between normal hearing people. We take this fact so much for granted that when a partner's hearing is affected we go through a gamut of reactions. Deafness is an irritating handicap requiring more work and consideration from the hearing partner. There is unlikely to be anyone in the family able to explain why the deaf person can hear some things and not others; why he appears disorientated, is sometimes sick and giddy by turns; complains of peculiar noises in his head; and, although fitted with an expensive hearing aid, still fails to understand. There may be a fear of travel due to the possible muddles of wrong train, wrong place, wrong time, and it must be remembered that telephoning is not possible if the deaf person is stranded.

For the hearing partner, there is no denying that the daily round without the stimulus of idle chat, exchange of ideas and news, and the odd joke, becomes boring. A state of despondency and unhappiness may set in on both sides unless help is available to show the hearing partner exactly what to expect, and what she can do to alleviate distress and eruptions at home. Where the home situation had already deteriorated before the onset of deafness, then matters are made worse and may lead to an additional excuse for divorce or separation.

Whenever possible, the most profitable answer is for the hearing person to accompany the deaf adult to a seminar or class and be made fully aware of the difficulties that the latter will now face. Understanding the consequences of a hearing loss, and what may be done to alleviate frustrations at home, is half the battle to deal with the future for both sides.

It should be obvious that the speaker would be better to wait until the deaf adult came face to face rather than try to shout upstairs or out to the kitchen for him.

It should be obvious that a deaf person cannot look down at his plate and continue to lipread — it may mean that chat has to wait until after a meal.

A hearing partner has to accept that the deaf person needs to withdraw at times. Lipreading is a great strain and until a degree of skill is reached there is much confusion, so that the lipreader requires periods of rest. Because of this I would advocate that the hearing partner keeps her own hobbies or occupations going, so that both sides are refreshed when they are together again.

The most successful rehabilitations I have seen have been where both partners are aware of what stresses and strains will now be put on a marriage and make a determined effort to work at easing the situation. For the hearing partner it means constantly remembering the communication problem and resorting to pencil and paper as a sensible alternative. For the deaf partner it means remembering that life has become more restricted and less easy for the hearing person. Neither should use the handicap as a recrimination or as an excuse.

There are practical points to consider. It may benefit both sides to have an adaptor for the television that will amplify sound for the deaf and enable the hearing person to keep to the normal sound level. There is a telephone amplifier to enable those with a reasonable loss to use the telephone still. There are systems, such as Ceefax and Teletext, which may be bought to enable the deaf to keep abreast of news and other items of interest. It may be useful to both to have a loop system installed in the house, and other items such as flashing lights to replace doorbells, alarm clocks with a low-tone bell, vibrating pillows to help a worker wake on time, and amplifiers for use between partners that are more powerful, albeit larger, than the individual aid. Some of these things are available through the Social Services, others by contacting the Royal National Institute for the Deaf, and others through commercial firms. Addresses are given at the end of the book (pages 234–6).

I remember with sadness one gentleman saying to me, after his wife's deafness had been diagnosed, 'I feel that we've both lost something from our lives. I've always thought that "marriages are made in Heaven" but I see now that on earth they are based on the delights of communication and that has been taken from us.' I had every hope that they would regain their conversational pleasures in time, because the wife was a sterling character who would tackle new difficulties with fervour and he would be supportive throughout.

I dislike a sentimental attitude and approach towards any form of handicap. To face it as fact, accept the limitations it imposes, and work at alleviating these as much as possible seems to be a worthwhile task. A common remark heard from the deaf themselves, as well as from workers in the field, is that there is a lack of understanding in the public attitude towards the deaf.

This is true, but training is needed if people are to be made aware of all the ramifications of the effects of not being able to hear. Also before attaching blame to other people it is as well to ponder the very real difficulties that deafness poses for others, and this must begin within the family unit for the ripples to spread outwards.

The elderly deaf

I shall hear in Heaven   Beethoven

It is very probable that the majority of the elderly deaf will also need to wait like Beethoven. It is possible throughout this book, to indicate what is required to alleviate the problems of a hearing loss but so much of all that is required is dependent upon the availability of trained personnel, the length of waiting lists and, for the elderly, the important factor of regular provision of transport. The elderly may not have too much time left to wait. When we reach our seventies, eighties, and nineties we have to accept and cope with the ageing process; there will be a slowing down of understanding and response although we know we have retained our mental faculties and, if we have a hearing loss, there will be a reduced ability to listen. Our physical inabilities are problems enough and if we are also treated as idiots because we cannot hear so well, then the easier and less degrading response is just to give up trying to listen. I have been told so often by elderly people that they 'are very deaf and can't hear a thing' when, in fact, they have stopped using their residual hearing and given up all attempts to concentrate. We all need some stimulation to listen — a particular voice, some interesting news, some gory details. We have all experienced shutting ourselves off from a boring lecturer either because we cannot hear his voice too well or because his delivery is dull.

Beethoven had no opportunity to use any electronic hearing aids and, as his museum at Bonn bears witness, he desperately tried the whole gamut of aids available in his day, mainly variations on the ear trumpet. Finally, he must have become too severely deaf to make use of these, since we are told that he composed his last work by vibrating a tuning fork held between his teeth to 'feel' the notes. However, the ear trumpet is still a very suitable aid for the elderly. It does not require a battery, there is no interference to create distortion, no special mould is required and it is easy to handle. It works on the same principle as the speaking tube used by a ship's captain sending orders to his crew. It provides very good amplification of high quality and, frequently, an elderly person who is unable to use a hearing aid can understand well with a speaking tube.

The small hearing aids worn behind the ear are far from easy for arthritic fingers to adjust. I found that in nine out of ten homes which I would visit the small aid always had to be unearthed from a drawer. It had either been too difficult for the wearer to adjust or instructions had been forgotten or never fully understood. Sometimes the owner saw little need to wear it when he was on his own for most of the week.

The larger bodyworn aid is more suitable. The controls of this are visible when worn and can more easily be adjusted. Visitors can hold the aid a short distance from their faces and speak with a moderate voice directly into the microphone or, alternatively, the aid can be placed on a table between them. A long lead is available for this purpose and can be asked for at issue or supplied from the audiology department of a hospital.

Problems for the elderly are compounded by the fact that not only are they hard of hearing but the sensation of loudness is also disturbed. If a sound is too loud it may be so unpleasant that it can even be painful, although to the normal person it would not seem so. The tolerance level may be very low so it is important not to shout. It is unlikely that the elderly will hear high notes very well, if at all, so they should watch the speaker's face to give them the best understanding. Many elderly people do not do this — they potter about the room while you are speaking or rummage for something they wish to show you — and it is important that you indicate that you will talk when they are looking at you. It is usually the start of a sentence that is missed, especially if the subject is unfamiliar, because the listener is not ready for it. It therefore saves time, and is less wearing, to make a short introduction e.g. 'I'm going to talk about my holiday'; then to start your conversation.

For the very elderly it is their privilege and often the easiest way for them to opt out of the difficulties of conversing. They have no job in jeopardy and if they have found that other people are irritated by their slowness and impatient at the need for repetition, then they are likely to give up making any effort, so that many aids which have been issued are left unused for want of a little training and perseverance. Thus the lonely become even more lonely. Should an elderly person be able to attend a lipreading group — and I have known ninety-year-old class members — then the sympathetic attitude found there and the advice and practice given become wonderful stimulants. However, the approach can be difficult. The words 'class' and 'lipreading' may well indicate to the elderly the problems of other people to cope with and something new to learn. This is not to say that the elderly will not benefit from lipreading classes but perhaps they should go under another title to make them appear less academic.

This may be a suitable place to note the problems that arise if and when a deaf person is in hospital or has to spend time in a nursing home. A Hospital Staff Guide is available from the main British Deaf Associations but it is doubtful whether every new nurse or doctor will have read it. For any deaf person a stay in hospital can be a nerve-shattering experience. They may be left in a world of smiles and nods but in total ignorance from which there is no escape. Their inability to communicate brings confusion and embarrassment. They can be left out of the general chat in the ward and feel isolated from their fellow patients. Sometimes their hearing aid is left at home or tucked into Sister's drawer.

It should be a routine matter to ask on admittance whether a patient is hard of hearing or totally deaf; and what sort of hearing aid they have. Then this information can be attached to papers on the bed. Some profoundly deaf people with a longstanding deafness may have defective speech and then it would be helpful to add the name of a relative who can communicate with them. I appreciate that professional staff may not have the time to sit and converse or write down messages for the deaf patient but hospitals have visitors, such as Friends of the Hospital, who could be advised that a deaf person needs befriending.

To summarize

Allow the elderly to settle and sit comfortably; eliminate distractions.

Talk face to face, at the same level, making certain that the speaker's face is in a good light.

Talk clearly in a moderately loud voice and do not shout.

Reduce the speed of your own speech. Leave longer intervals between sentences.

Check that any hearing aid is working either by listening through it yourself or going through a few numbers to see if the wearer can repeat these to you.

Hold the aid in hand if possible and keep the microphone towards the speaker.

If you are a regular visitor to the deaf then invest in an ear trumpet to take with you. I well recall having a Danish lady in one class who had been issued with two excellent post-aural aids but who found these very difficult to put into her ears and adjust. When I suggested that she should buy an ear trumpet, she found it so successful that she carried it home triumphantly, no doubt boasting at the acquisition of her 'new British hearing aid!'

2

WHAT HAPPENS

Why is this thus? What is the reason for this thusness?
Artemus Ward (American humorist)

Causes of Deafness

Not knowing the cause of their deafness can be a worry to some deaf people. Obviously if one knows that there is an heredity factor, or has recovered from an acute illness such as meningitis, or is now elderly, then a cause is apparent. Others are informed by specialists that a serious accident has damaged one working part of the ear. I say one *working* part because the external ear seems to be of little use in modern man other than to act as a dust-trap — its directional abilities no longer apply, although most of us have met the man who can still wiggle his ears at a party. Van Gogh might have been unbalanced enough to cut off his ear but this would not have affected his hearing ability.

Functionally the ear has two paths. First, there is a perceiving apparatus which begins in the hair cells of the inner ear and ends in the primary and psychic auditory areas of the brain. Secondly, a conducting apparatus consisting of the ear-drum, a chain of small bones to relay the vibrations from the drum, the middle ear cleft, and the fluid of the inner ear. Either one or both of these parts may suffer damage or be almost totally destroyed and, in many cases a cause is unknown.

There is a condition, called otosclerosis in which the hard, mature bones of the ear are replaced with a soft, spongy bone, usually on the promontory in front of the oval window leading to the inner ear. This condition spreads until the small bones are, in fact, bolted down and can no longer move freely to transmit sound vibrations. In such cases surgery is often possible and after a successful operation these patients receive maximum benefit from a hearing aid.

A particular ear condition, known as Ménière's syndrome, causes a hearing loss associated with intermittent attacks of severe vertigo and tinnitus. Such attacks are misery for the sufferers, who are often unable to stand for several days at a time. I have had a client who performed her household tasks on her knees during such attacks, which may often disappear for years and then recur without warning.

Hearing may be lowered by chronic catarrh which, if persistent, can produce a swelling of the Eustachian tube, which connects the middle ear with the throat. The purpose of the tube is to provide ventilation and drainage for the middle ear and to equalize air pressure on both sides of the eardrum. Infections can cause a fluctuation in the hearing, which may clear with treatment. Throat infections may also involve the ear by way of the Eustachian tube: when the tube swells and closes, and the middle ear is filled with fluid, there is a feeling of stuffiness and the pressure may reach a point where the ear-drum bursts and the fluid drains out into the ear canal. A running ear should never be taken lightly, nor should any attempt be made to remove a foreign body from your own or another person's ear. In most people there is a 'waist' in the canal which narrows at a point about halfway back to the drum and then becomes larger again. It is a delicate task to dig out any substance, especially if it is a hard object, and it should be left for the doctor to deal with.

Other common causes of infection include diseased tonsils and sinuses, and frequent and heavy colds. The toxins of meningitis, scarlet fever, mumps, syphilis, and the like, if carried to the inner ear by the blood, or entering the fluid that fills it, may destroy some of the delicate nerve endings. Traumatic accidents such as falling from a height, being knocked from a cycle, or being hit on the head by a hard object, may all cause severe deafness.

Within recent years it has been my experience that causes of deafness due to massive drug intake are on the increase. Modern surgical skills can give a person a new kidney but, in the course of treatment, heavy drug dosage may be required which destroys the nerves of the inner ear. I do not use the word 'destroys' lightly, because one consequence has been, in the clients I have met, that no vestige of vibration remains. Because these clients have been rendered totally deaf overnight, individual lipreading sessions are essential and speech conservation is usually necessary to retain a fairly normal pattern of speech. In an effort to use vibration to instil a sense of the rhythmic nature of a phrase or sentence, it has been found that the deaf client is unable to feel the vibration of a telephone when his hand is placed on a ringing instrument or to feel the chords of a piano when he is standing behind with his hands resting on the frame. This is most unusual and means resorting to a tactile method of placing hands on chest, throat and jawbone, as one would need to do with the deaf-blind.

Deafness caused by ototoxicity is not new. The first known reported case may be that of the Duke of Wellington. In 1822, when the Duke was fifty-three years old, he was treated by a 'quack specialist' who tried to cure his deafness by syringeing his ear with a strong caustic solution. Afterwards the Duke noticed that his hearing was very sensitive; he said that the noise of a carriage passing along the street was like the loudest thunder and that anyone who spoke to him seemed to be shrieking at the top of his voice. When he was seen by Dr Hume, a medical man who had been at Waterloo, the doctor noticed that he staggered like a drunken man.

It has long been recognized that many drugs are powerful enough to cause toxic damage, for example quinine, arsenic, and alcohol. But it is often difficult to establish cause and effect in such cases. To begin with, patients receive many drugs to take either singly or in combination at one time and the effects do not always begin immediately nor do they stop after taking the drug; also, it is difficult to experiment clinically because of danger to the patient. The hearing impairment that accompanies ototoxicity is always senso-neural and may be temporary, following the use of the salicylates, quinine or strong diuretics, or it may be permanent as in the case of heavy metals.

Doctors receive Adverse Drug Reaction Bulletins, which

give information on drug-induced deafness, and the list of the mycin drugs is especially alarming. A study of the different ototoxic mechanisms involved has already yielded interesting insights into the nature of the deafness itself, and we must remember that patients undergoing vital operations have little chance of survival without the use of drugs in their treatment and recovery. No doubt the number of such drug-induced deaf patients is still relatively small, but perhaps a forewarning is indicated to prepare such patients for the additional trauma of deafness which they are likely to have to face.

There are known cases of hysterical deafness, which require careful handling, where a course of individual lipreading, followed by a group session, is often necessary. Neither should one take amiss the remark of one anxious lady who, when asked if she knew the cause of her deafness, said that it stemmed from the day on which she had been caught by her father with her ear at the door of his study.

Where the cause is known, an explanation can be given if required; otherwise time is wasted trying to find 'a reason for this thusness' and clients should be led to see this, so that there is little delay in starting a programme of rehabilitation.

Tinnitus

> The bells of hell go ting-a-ling-aling, For you and not for me.
>
>   (Song of 1914–18 war)

I might say this to a tinnitus sufferer. Although it is not strictly accurate because, although head noises have been designated with the term tinnitus (from the Latin for bell), ringing is but one of the great variety of noises endured by sufferers. Roget's Thesaurus has ten sections on words to describe sound from sound in general, to others denoting loudness, through specific sounds of burst, explosion and backfire, to words for resonance, cries and animal sounds. It seems to me that, at one time or another, all these words have been used by tinnitus sufferers in an effort to describe to me the noises they experience in their head.

The condition of tinnitus is not always allied to a loss of hearing. Many sufferers have normal hearing but, naturally, trying to hear people over an inner, frantic sound does not help one to appear alert and sensible nor make one wish to be especially sociable. How much worse, therefore, when a sufferer from head noises also endures a hearing loss and has two disabilities to cope with. Many times have I heard the remark from a tinnitus sufferer, 'If only I was just deaf!' since it is the constant internal noises which are so debilitating. One client said to her husband, 'I had always assumed that being deaf meant being in a silent world, not a noisier one,' for that is how it must seem if you hear bells ringing all the time you are awake, or steamrollers rumbling down stretches of road, or a swishing sound, or waves breaking.

I now think of tinnitus in a visual form as akin to the famous painting by Edvard Munch called The Scream, in which the dreadful open mouth externalizes the noise. I imagine that tinnitus sufferers have an internalized scream that is worse than any silence, which can have them waking, shaking, in the night. It is difficult to imagine and it is difficult to see how sufferers can possibly manage the everyday matter of living by rising above it — and I am not exaggerating. Just speak with a sufferer for a few minutes and you will understand their suicidal feelings. Naturally, there are degrees of the problem, as there are degrees of hearing loss; those who do not have it continuously, or who are able to subjugate it by external means, manage to hold their jobs and live with it.

No one seems quite to know what tinnitus is. When we were young, on holiday at the seaside, we would pick up a shell, hold it to our ear and say, 'I hear the sea.' What we were listening to were the sounds inside our bodies — after all, if sound is energy, then the workings of the heart, the circulation of the blood, even breathing, must cause noise and we all know that in quiet surroundings, when we are thinking of little else, we hear our own heartbeat. Perhaps the deaf person, with no external distraction, is forced to suffer these noises of his own making, although this does not explain the variety and volume of the descriptions given by deaf people. Very small abnormalities in the nerves of hearing can generate sounds of their own which are inaudible to other people and it is thought that in some types of tinnitus, the nerve cells, particularly the hair cells in the cochlea or inner ear, are in an excitable state. Several years of research have gone into trying to discover what it is that sufferers do hear and it is now possible to simulate these noises on a machine.

From these studies and experiments come forms of relief for some people. A person who is not totally deaf can use a masker. This is a small aid, rather like a hearing aid worn behind the ear, that will produce a sound louder than that heard inside the head. Before maskers were available, a sufferer would often hold a radio close to the ear, even in bed, in an effort to drown the internal noise. A tinnitus masker is basically a noise generator which feeds sound into the ear and, for those who have a hearing loss, it is possible to combine the masker with the hearing aid. However, working with sound is not as simple as working with vision. Whereas it is an easy matter to cover a windowframe with a piece of tape, and hide the frame completely, it is much more difficult to make a masker that will cover a spectrum of sounds. And, of course, those with a total hearing loss can gain no benefit at all from wearing one.

Unfortunately, it is still true to say that sufferers have to learn to 'live with' tinnitus. Some people are still told that they are imagining their noises, others have been referred for psychiatric treatment. But it *is* true to say that many sufferers find that the noises lessen if they can absorb themselves fully in work or a hobby. An actor says that he is never aware of his tinnitus on stage, or during rehearsals, but as soon as a performance is ended, the noises return. A lipreader will say that he is able to 'lose' his tinnitus while concentrating in a class and others have spoken of being free from their noises when able to lead a full and active life. For the majority, the noises are a permanent fixture of existence. Sometimes the sounds appear to have a more orderly structure — some people hear 'tinnitus music', others recognize familiar songs, or connected words and even sentences, so that one wonders whether part of the brain is not involved, if only in personal interpretations of the noises heard.

The British Tinnitus Association
In July 1979 the British Tinnitus Association was formed, with the aim of pooling the experiences of tinnitus

sufferers, both those with and without a hearing loss, and enable them to meet locally to exchange views, as well as becoming a catalyst towards finding a cure. A cure has not yet been found, but the Association is of great benefit to those who wish to meet other sufferers and the regular newsletter published by the RNID enables queries to be answered and suggestions to be circulated to all members. Initially it is a relief to find that you are not going mad, and that there are thousands of others experiencing similar disturbances, and those who do wish to talk over their feelings, or pass on anything they found which helped give relief, find the local meetings a bright spot in their lives.

Remedies

In desperation and ignorance many remedies have been tried — herbal cigarettes, vitamin tablets, cotton wool in the ears, hypnosis, acupuncture — and many sufferers are unable to get any respite from their noises without taking some brand of sleeping tablet. Tablets are given medically, since many tinnitus sufferers have mild depression and alleviation of the depression may help them to cope with the tinnitus itself, although the tablets will not affect the level of the tinnitus. From my experience, it is those who suffer a total loss, due in some degree to drug treatment for an illness, who have tinnitus to the greatest degree. They receive no outside stimulation to take their minds from the internalized noises, but it would also appear that there has been grave damage to the nerve endings in the ear.

For those needing to concentrate wholly on lipreading the noises are an added tribulation, and it is usually necessary to spend time talking about their tinnitus before any attempts can be made to improve a lipreading skill. One client said that she felt she was 'getting on top' of her noises by trying to become interested in them. She felt less worked up about them, and less worn out, if she made herself listen and try to interpret and then talk about them. If she could externalize the noise imaginatively, by following the steamroller she heard, up and down the road, then she felt more ready to push it literally into the back of her mind and deal with everyday matters. The noises never disappeared but she was able to make them take a back seat. If others find this an impossibility, then they are likely to become more and more isolated and unsociable.

At present, then, sufferers must try to find their own way of living with their noises until a cure is found. It seems pointless to start treating symptoms until the underlying pathology of the complaint is discovered. If tinnitus is the result of damage in the auditory apparatus then no drug can be expected to result in a cure. But work goes on: the Medical Research Council is a Government-funded body involved in tinnitus research projects, including various aspects of diagnosis and treatment; some universities are engaged in the investigation of cochlea ototoxicity in animals, or making detailed studies of the factors relevant to tinnitus; and the British Tinnitus Association distributes its latest findings through its bi-monthly newsletter. To help themselves, sufferers are advised to join the BTA, seek expert medical advice and try a tinnitus masker. Some people have been helped by joining a yoga class; reducing stress certainly helps people to cope better. I have also known a client, with intermittent tinnitus, receive relief from a course of acupuncture; but the response to treatment may have been coincidental since others have found no relief from similar treatment.

For people working in noisy conditions in industry, or who are otherwise exposed to prolonged periods of loud noise, such as gunfire, tinnitus is preventable if ear protection is worn. Anyone who works with noisy tools and experiences ringing in the ear should accept this as a warning sign and wear ear mufflers or wax inserts as protection.

Some people, reading the literature on the subject, think they are suffering from tinnitus because they have become extremely sensitive to loud sounds, amplified music, the noise from household appliances and car noises. But they are suffering from a condition called recruitment, which is common in ears that have a hearing loss. One solution is to wear ear plugs to reduce the sound level or special hearing aids are available which stop loud sounds reaching the ear.

Many people are desperately keen to pinpoint the cause of their tinnitus, but this does not make any treatment that may be available any more effective. Sufferers from Ménière's Disease, which is a condition consisting of deafness, vertigo with vomiting, and tinnitus, are usually given a drug to relieve the sickness and imbalance but which has little effect on the tinnitus, and those who have had an unsuccessful stapedectomy operation suffer tinnitus of the worst kind. But in all cases it is necessary to find an ENT specialist who will endeavour to pinpoint the cause of your tinnitus and prescribe a masker or a drug to alleviate the noises when they become unbearable. This is short-term relief until the happy day when a permanent cure has been found.

It is heartbreaking to have a deaf member of the family who also suffers from tinnitus because, although there are simple ways to help the lipreader, we can do nothing for the noises in the head. I cannot forget the episode related to me by a woman, totally deafened in middle age, who has such severe tinnitus that, despite a loving and under-standing husband, there are times when she wants to die. She had to become an in-patient at a local hospital to receive a hip replacement and woke one night — as she had done many times at home — with the tinnitus screaming in her head. She thinks she must have called out because the nurses came running, to find her sitting on the edge of the bed, holding her head in her hands. They sent for the doctor on call and when he came and was told that her tinnitus was unbearable, he took the woman by the shoulders, hugged her sypathetically and said that, even as a doctor, there was nothing he could do for her. Such episodes urge anyone who encounters a sufferer, or sufferers themselves, to join together to pool knowledge and press for funds to hasten research and the imperative need for a cure tomorrow — not in the next century.

Cochlear Implants

'What a blessing it would be if we could open and shut our ears as easily as we do our eyes.'
(Georg Lichtenberg, German physicist)

This thought, although first written down at the end of the eighteenth century, is now becoming a possibility at last. For almost ten years work has been in progress towards the development of a particular form of cochlear implant for the totally deaf. Many papers have been presented in this country, at meetings of the British Society of Audiology in

London, and exciting work is continuing to improve techniques and, evaluate results to assess the value of the implants and their future.

The idea of treating deafness by re-educative methods is not new, although until the advancement in surgical techniques actual implants were not possible. As early as 1802 Itard in France found out that, by repeated stimulation of the ear by a definite sound, the auditory sensibility increased. He used musical instruments to give his patients a sense of the direction of the sound and a sense of rhythm. He then proceeded in the same way with the voice, bombarding his pupils with vowels and consonants until they obtained some measure of improvement in their hearing. His methods lapsed for many years, until the end of the nineteenth century when a Dr Zund-Burguet of Paris invented an approach using what he termed 'the electrophonoide method' of stimulating the ear. This seems to have been the forerunner of what we now term an auditory trainer, which can reproduce the sound vibrations of the whole range of the human voice. Dr Zund-Burguet also claimed that his machine could produce a gentle disturbance of air which would lend a 'vibratory massage' to the middle and external ears and the tickling sensation was found most agreeable by his patients.

Deafness is by no means a newcomer among the many afflictions of humanity; Moses declared, 'Thou shalt not curse the deaf,' but until less than two hundred years ago deafness caused by wax was the only form of deafness that was treated. An early aural surgeon is quoted as saying, 'There are two kinds of deafness — the one is due to wax and is curable and the other is not due to wax and is not curable.' I was also interested to find that the mild-mannered Dr Hawley Harvey Crippen had a connection with deafness. A firm called Aural Remedies Company had premises in Craven House, Kingsway, in London. They advertised a treatment for deafness 'on the lines of the late Drouet Institute' and said that they had, as consultant, one H.H. Crippen M.D., a graduate of an American Homoeopathic Hospital College, who was at one time connected with the Drouet Institute and 'has also been interested in other quack remedies'!

This seems to have been the position before the advent of

hearing aids. The first instruments were bulky and cumbersome, in fact for many people the physical pressures of the aid must have distracted them from the benefits. There was also disappointment that perception through the instrument was not as good as natural hearing, but fears that wearing an aid would make the user dependent on the device or thoughts that, if he laid it aside, his hearing would be worse than before, were quite unfounded. However, all these methods were applied externally, even though sounds were actually transmitted to the inner ear in order to stimulate nerve endings.

In 1800 it was reported that Alessandro Volta (the physicist for whom the volt was named) was brave enough to place a rod electrode into his own ears and turn on an electric current. He said that he heard a sound 'like thick boiling soup', and that must have been one of the earliest experiments with electrical stimulation of the auditory system.

However, in the late 1950s two otologists made the first attempt to place electrodes in the inner ear (the cochlea) to stimulate it actively. By 1975 the results on the first few patients they had done enthused others and an American team began implanting four patients in Oklahoma in 1978, stating that if the results were successful, the project would be continued and broadened, if unsuccessful, they would stop and report those failings. They took adults who were profoundly deaf, had no ear infection and who had good lipreading ability and intelligible speech. Despite a few initial failures, due to some physical rejection of the implanted coil, results showed that the door to inner ear deafness was opening.

I find it interesting that the otologists were surprised that many of their candidates for implants rejected the idea out of hand. These people had a chronic personal fear, not so much of the operation involved but because of sudden anxiety about future responsibilities if they had to compete in a world of sound, after having lived for so many years in a world without it.

The principal advantage of the cochlear implant so far has been to increase the patient's ability to hear environmental sounds. The implant usually makes it possible for the user to hear these sounds at a level much closer to that at which a normal hearing person would hear them. For example, a deaf person, using a hearing aid, may only hear a telephone if he is very close to it. With the implant he can hear it from a greater distance, and similarly with a doorbell and other household noises. As yet, patients have gained only very limited speech understanding but they can hear their own voices and therefore are able to monitor their own voices better. They can tell the difference between a man and a woman's voice, but they describe speech as sounding very distorted or muffled. What does seem a worthwhile improvement is the fact that lipreading is improved. People with the implants receive more clues from the sounds and rhythms of speech, and can often distinguish voiced from unvoiced sounds, which helps to iron out some of the homophenous problems.

However, if a deaf person is already an accomplished lipreader then to undergo an implant would require serious weighing of the advantages. Becoming a cochlear implant patient is an involved business. Apart from suitability as regards age and hearing loss, there are many preliminary tests to undergo; the implant surgery would require at least a few days in hospital; and rehabilitation and training in the use of the implant involves several months of training, involving family members.

Those patients who have received the cochlear implant are greatly encouraged because they 'hear' the sound within their head. They say they feel more in contact with the world about them; that they can hear the mood in people's voices; they can 'hear' excitement and happiness, so that these new auditory sensations obviously increase their awareness of surroundings and are an aid to communication. When the physical properties and complications of high frequency tones are overcome, then it would certainly benefit all deaf people to be able to hear the high consonants once more, since this would increase tonotopic information and enable them to understand language.

Undoubtedly cochlear implant surgery will continue to improve over the years. There will be more complex instruments and better devices developed to improve speech communication, and work in this country is being supported by the Medical Research Council. But research and clinical trials are very costly and time consuming, so it may be many years before the widespread application of cochlear implants can become a reality for the great majority of deaf persons.

3

THE HEARING AID AND
AUDITORY TRAINING

O precious bane
Tormenting joy,
Dividing chain,
Exacting toy.

This oxymoron, although originally descriptive of the telephone, may well be used as a description of a hearing aid. I do not intend to deal with the mechanics of a hearing aid (although some suggestions will be made as to its care and maintenance), but rather to deal with the use of an aid as well as its limitations. The majority of hearing aid users will admit that they had little initial advice as to what they might expect of their device, that it was not easy to get used to wearing it, or the new sounds heard from it, but that they would not or could not be without one.

I have known only two hearing aid users, in my years of working with adults, who were able to have their aids fitted and depart joyfully. Both had a partial loss spread evenly over all frequencies and, once the aid was fitted, were able to receive sound almost normally again. But few hearing losses are like this and not many wearers can be given an aid which is completely suited to the particular hearing loss present, although much time is given to matching the performance of an aid to an individual loss as closely as possible, and the range of aids available through the National Health Service has been greatly increased in recent years.

In the early days hearing aids were issued after the diagnosis of a hearing loss using pure tone sound tests. Teachers of deaf children have always been aware that it is of greater importance to know what sounds of speech a child can still receive, in order either to correct mispronunciations or to teach the sound through another medium, such as vision or touch. It has now been realized that adults also need to be given a speech discrimination test. As human beings we are able to recognize the differences between various things: we don't walk into a door because we see it is different from the walls; and we don't eat food with a disagreeable smell. With each of our senses we are able to discriminate among many things which stimulate a particular sense. Imagine what it would be like if you could not discriminate between the vowel sounds of the English language — regardless of whether the speaker said a,e,i,o or u, you would hear the same sound. This would clearly be a considerable handicap and it would be an even greater handicap if your vowel discrimination was unimpaired but your ability to discriminate consonants were faulty. So that although pure tone tests have been and still are very valuable it is now recognized that this provides rather limited information about a person's ability to hear the most numerous and significant sounds to which he is exposed — the sounds of speech.

The customary method of measuring the listener's speech discrimination is to determine the percentage of words he can hear and repeat correctly, when they are presented to him at a comfortable loudness. After a pure tone test the listener will be told that, 'this will now be a test of your ability to hear words. Instead of whistles and humming sounds you will hear a recording of a man talking and when he tells you to say a word, say that word out loud. If you think you know a word but aren't quite sure, don't be afraid to guess.' And so a result is arrived at which will enable the audiologist to select a more suitable aid. Tests may also be given for auditory recruitment.

There are people with a conductive or middle ear deafness who find they can hear conversation perfectly well when they are in noisy places. But if they listen in the quiet, without a hearing aid, these same persons will be at a disadvantage unless the speaker raises his voice and speaks very loudly. In other words, listeners of this kind are aided rather than disturbed by loud sounds. By way of contrast, many persons with nerve deafness cannot tolerate noisy places. You will be familiar with those with an inner ear deafness who obviously do not understand when you speak in a normal voice but who will say, when you raise your voice to help them, 'Don't shout, I'm not deaf'. These people are demonstrating one aspect of auditory recruitment — poor tolerance for loud sounds. These differences indicate the importance of thorough testing to learn as much as possible about the individual's hearing loss.

How to Get a Hearing Aid

If a person suspects he has a hearing loss then a visit to a local doctor is the first step. The GP may find wax in the ear, or an infection, and after these are treated the hearing may improve and no further visit is necessary. However, if the hearing is still poor, or is not due to wax, then there will be a referral to the ENT (Ear, Nose and Throat) department of a hospital for more specialized examination. Medical or surgical treatment may be necessary and if the hearing is still poor then the patient will be sent to the Hearing Aid Centre. There an impression for an ear mould will be taken. When this is ready — which may be a matter of weeks — then a hearing aid is fitted. An appointment will be given for a follow-up check, and instructions given as to control of the parts on the aid and on repairs.

Unless the hospital has a hearing therapist on its audiological team there is no likelihood of the wearer of the aid being offered training sessions in its use. No practical help is given with the problem of the disorientation that can arise from the absence of ambient noise, or its misinterpretation. The inability to decipher the cacophony of sounds in crowded places leads to an odd sense of unreality and of not being with the world. This is heightened if there is any suggestion of an unexpected event, such as an accident, because of the inability to locate something happening at a distance or to sense the mood of a crowd.

Information Through Hearing

It is a revelation to discover just how much information our hearing provides in everyday life. Apart from listening to what people say, we hear the water boiling, bacon frying, the doorbell and the clock, someone coming up behind us, the radio humming, and although it is easy to see that it is windy or raining, the force of both are assessed aurally — a breeze and a gale may look the same but they certainly sound different. The sense of hearing is truly directional — we look immediately to the spot where we have dropped something; we can locate keys at the bottom of a bag without looking; we can identify footsteps and monitor events in all directions. Lack of hearing can lead to inappropriate actions, such as looking for people in the wrong part of the house, bumping into people, and a general clumsiness. It is not hard to realize that understanding of speech is not the only difficulty involved in a hearing loss, and any lipreading skill will only take us so far. How much greater use it would be if we could combine a set of aural clues with the visual ones received in watching faces, and if we knew just when it would be wise to keep our hearing aid on and when it might prove less harrowing to switch it off.

Then, too, through our aid we are hearing sound as we never heard it before. How can we recognize and identify the new noises, especially if we have been growing deaf over a number of years, now have a powerful aid, and are in the position of a blind man regaining partial sight and not recognizing what it is he sees? All-round rehabilitation must, therefore, include not only counselling when an aid is issued, lipreading tuition to encourage and improve visual skill, but also auditory training periods to enable the hearing aid user to discriminate sounds and, where indicated, voice conservation.

Few of us listen intently all the time — just as we do not take in a complete picture with our sight at first glance. Unless we are deeply interested in a subject a part of our thoughts is on other things; but hearing people can still take in enough to understand the theme of a conversation or lecture. When we really mean to listen with our full concentration we say, 'I'm all ears' or 'You have my full attention' and then we do try to listen to every word. Those with a hearing loss need to concentrate hard *all the time* in order to add an aural clue to the visual and to give their mind the best possible chance to interpret.

Many deaf people can actually hear more than they think they can. Even tested with a simple balanced word list —

which eliminates contextual guidance — they are often astonished that they have been able to make even a reasonable score. Then, when shown the hearing 'errors' it makes more sense to be told that it would be worth their while attempting to retrain the ear, to endeavour to distinguish sounds through the aid, in an effort to increase speech comprehension.

At the present time most hearing aid users attempt to use their new aid by the inefficient method of trial and error, since no one has taken the responsibility to explain the principles of amplification and how to use the aid beneficially. This can lead to dissatisfaction with the aid and recrimination against either the National Health Service or the private agent.

A point to remember is that no hearing aid is superior to the normal hearing mechanism. As the name implies, an aid is designed to help the wearer hear sounds; it does not correct an auditory disorder. Therefore, the benefits derived from an aid depend on accurate evaluation in the first place and the willingness of the wearer to accept its limitations. If, then, training is given in correct usage, using the residual hearing to the full in an attempt to recognize distorted speech, the hearing aid user will gain maximum benefit from a most useful instrument. I am still surprised how many users will push a piece of plastic into an ear, fiddle with controls that are out of sight and say, 'I don't know that it does much for me'. Surely, not only the wearer but all the family should know what the aid is capable of doing, so that dishes are not banged about in the presence of a hearing aid wearer, television and stereo controls are not turned up suddenly, nor the wearer expected to respond from another room just because he is wearing 'an aid to hearing'.

The Components of a Hearing Aid

Before discussing what material is useful for listening practice it is as well to be familiar with the components of an aid. I have found that many users have little idea of the name or the function of each part. This is not necessarily because they have never been told. We must remember that anyone attending a Centre, to be fitted with an aid, may be in a nervous state, unable to lipread and, of course, until the aid is fitted and working properly, unable to hear instructions properly.

The part which will receive most use is the *volume* or *gain control*. This is what makes the input signals louder or softer. The wearer should be told how to position this when his hearing loss is evaluated. At the same time he should understand how to adjust the control in varying circumstances, that is, in a quiet room, in traffic, or indoors. Usually the aid will operate most effectively when it is between one-quarter and three-quarters on, but new wearers tend to have the aid tuned too low because they are not used to amplified sound and find it abnormally loud at first.

The *battery* is the heart of the aid. Without one the aid will not work, so its condition is critical. The wearer needs to know how to insert a new battery and take out the spent one, the type and size of replacement required, and the proper storage of spares. An over-sized battery can damage the housing of the battery compartment because it is forced in, and an under-sized battery will not fit properly nor make proper contact, so that reception might be intermittent. If batteries are bought in a batch of half a dozen then unused ones should be kept in a dry, cool place.

The *ear mould* both holds the aid in the wearer's ear and conducts the sounds into it from the receiver of the aid. The mould should fit snugly and feel comfortable inside the ear. If the fit is loose, or the mould not correctly inserted, this will result in the amplified sound being fed back to the outside air, resulting in a squeal or whistling sound.

Some aids have a *tone control*, similar to those on radios, stereos and television receivers. This allows the wearer to adjust the *quality* of the sound, that is, it can give emphasis to low frequencies (bass) or high frequencies (treble). This should not be confused with the volume control and normally is kept at the same setting that it was on when the aid was fitted.

An accessory of the aid which is often misused is the *telephone pick-up coil*, marked as T on some aids but not all. When the control is switched on, the aid responds to magnetic variations within the telephone receiver rather than to sound pressure variations or acoustic energy. Therefore, when this switch is engaged the aid will amplify only sounds that are transmitted by the telephone receiver. This may well help a user who has to use a telephone in a noisy background. Just remember to disengage the T control after a telephone conversation or the aid will not function. Also, care must be taken in using the control; it is so easy to substitute one for another as they are positioned so closely. The switch may be put inadvertently to T rather than O for Off, which results in battery wastage.

The *plastic tubing* connecting the ear mould with the main body of the aid requires regular attention. It should be cut just long enough to enable the aid to sit comfortably behind the ear. Too short, and the aid will fall forward or rest uneasily high without support; too long, and the aid will 'waggle' and feel a constant nuisance. The tubing can dry and crack with use and in some climatic conditions. Since it is not too easy to fit a new piece without practice, a visit to the Audiology Centre for a replacement is the best solution. It is a pity that aids for adults were not fitted with the wire extension first made on the aids given to children, since this caused far fewer problems and was a better sound conductor.

On a body-worn aid there will be a lead instead of the plastic tubing. This is sometimes broken internally, particularly if it gets chewed and twisted, and so needs replacing; or the two connecting points may be broken and not fit exactly into the casing of the aid or the mould, so it is useful to have a spare at hand that you can exchange for the damaged one.

As may be seen, an aid needs to be fully understood to be appreciated and used to advantage. Ignorance is at the root of much dissatisfaction expressed by wearers and this could so easily be prevented by initial explanations.

Degrees of Hearing Loss

Hearing loss is measured in decibels, a decibel being the unit of sound measurement and 30–45 about equal to a whisper at three feet. Professionally, a hearing loss of *30–40 decibels* is a moderate loss affecting the scanning and background functions of hearing. It is the point at which conversation becomes difficult without some amplification. There is no problem with communication provided the speaker comes close but it is the impaired awareness of sound which is important.

A loss of *45–65 decibels* would mean that social intercourse is affected. Because background noises are lost, the response is only to foreground stimulation. Amplification is helpful for conversation but it needs to be limited to one person or a small group. This can lead to social detachment and a search to find other people with a similar degree of deafness.

A loss of *65–80 decibels* means that amplification is less satisfactory. Both personal and environmental contact is difficult. The adult needs to put a greater reliance on visual signals and becomes more dependent on lipreading.

A loss of *80–100 decibels* is a profound loss. Amplification is useful to help maintain personal speech and for focusing on loud sounds.

This is a fairly rough calculation because other factors, such as age of onset, personality, and education, must necessarily affect the ability with which a person can cope with his loss. Even so, the entire range of hearing loss can benefit from some attempt at auditory training. Those whose residual hearing, whether natural or amplified with an aid, enables them to be aware of acoustic stimuli can learn to improve their discrimination of sounds. As an example, one client may suffer a severe loss for high tones (the consonants) and a less severe loss for the low tones (the vowels). With the help of an aid she is able to amplify the sounds she hears to the extent of picking out some middle-range consonants; but the amplification of the low tones has not helped her to discriminate between the grosser vowels, and these sound very distorted to her, with little difference between the sounds of 'er' and 'or'. Not knowing what she actually hears of these sounds a teacher can only present words and sentences repetitively in the hope that the client will learn to recognize a difference if these are fed into her aid often enough. The fact that she recognizes that 'bird' does not sound the same as 'board' means she heard *something* dissimilar and, in time, she is able to recognize correctly such similarities as, 'The bird fell down/the board fell down'. This doesn't sound much until you think of the number of words which contain these two vowels and discover that the deaf are always muddling 'thirty' and 'forty' over the telephone.

Some letters consist of a number of sounds running together. For example, when we say the sound of the letter 'w' we are really making the sound of 'oo' plus the neutral 'a'. When said very quickly this comes out as 'wa' but we have actually used two frequencies. Since this same client could no longer hear the neutral 'a', she picked up only 'oo' so that words containing the sound of w were not recognized. When she was shown this her mind became orientated to the fact of the new w and the problem eased.

It certainly is such an interesting subject. I could say to a client, 'Can you hear this?' and repeat the soft sound of pa pa pa pa. 'No', he would say.

Well, what do you think this word is — ill. That is ill. Good.

Now, what do you think this word is — pill. Oh, that's pill.

This would indicate that he heard *something* for p but that it was obviously not recognizable in isolation and would be worth practice in listening to until it became familiar.

As it is not easy to find a professional able to give practice, what could you do for yourself?

Suggested exercises in attentiveness

1. Observe people whose voices are the most difficult or the easiest for you to understand. Try to think out why this is so.
    Note rooms and situations which you find difficult.

2. Find out the best distance at which you can follow conversation. Does this vary with the different voices in your family?

3. As you move from room to room try to identify consciously, sounds which are audible to you: a clock, outside traffic, water running, a plane overhead. Make it a habit to stop, look and listen.

4. Observe the moods of individuals or groups: can you identify humour, doubt, disapproval, concern, anger?

5. Begin to make a list of words which you find difficult. You can use the television for this, turning the volume to where you experience difficulty.

Sound Memory

One serious aspect of hearing loss is that lack of normal use and exercise for the hearing centres of the brain, over long periods of time, causes loss of sound memory. I know people who have been deaf for thirty or forty years who have forgotten common household sounds: they cannot remember what sound water made running from the tap, or a letterbox rattling, or a Hoover in action. You may wonder of what importance these sounds are, but it is environmental sounds like these which keep us aware of things going on about us and stimulate us.

Hold on to your memory of sound by practising lists of common words, either by saying five or six at a time out loud or asking a friend to say them to you and you repeat back. Then try increasing the speed of these.

If you can hear the radio, spend a few minutes every day listening to one sentence, turning off the sound and then seeing if you can repeat the entire sentence exactly as you heard it.

If a member of your family can make a tape for you then tape some of the common everyday sounds: someone coming downstairs; the telephone ringing, the front door bell; a sneeze; money falling on the ground; an alarm clock; a tap running; a door banging. Then try to listen and say what these are.

Tape some different musical sounds: a bit of piano music, the violin, drums, a trumpet, the cymbals, even the triangle. Listen and pick them out. Make a tape of different voices: listen to a man's voice, a woman's; children speaking, laughing and screaming; a lecturer; your own family's voices; singing.

Make a tape of outdoor sounds: lorries, cycles, buses, an aeroplane, the dustman, the milkman. Tape anything, to play occasionally, test yourself and keep your awareness.

Hearing Speech

The understanding of speech, of course, is of prime importance. The intensity level of speech is surprisingly small: our vocal cords can convert only a fraction of the air stream flowing from our lungs into acoustic energy. Also, when we speak, the sound energy is scattered in all directions. Even if we ask someone to speak steadily at a normal conversational level, the speech intensities vary greatly as the speaker produces sound after speech sound. The vowels are the strongest sounds, although there is still a wide range of intensity amongst these. The strongest vowel is aw, which is about three times as strong as ee. And whereas the strongest of the consonants, r, is about the same intensity as ee, it is quite two and a half times the strength of sh, six times as strong as n and 200 times stronger than the weakest consonant th. Therefore, unless speakers are standing fairly close, there will be many sounds without the intensity to carry very far.

Speech remains fully intelligible until its intensity becomes so high that it causes pain. But the threshold of pain varies in individuals, so that care should be taken in increasing volume too much on a hearing aid. When speech and noise are about equal then people hear about half of what is being said to them. But sometimes we are able to understand speech when its intensity is lower than that of noise, and this is because our perceptual mechanism somehow manages to separate the two — this helps us in a busy street, for example.

Many experiments have been performed with natural speech to find out which range of frequencies is essential for speech recognition. Devices have been made that respond only to certain frequencies, which can filter out the others, so that we are able to listen to sentences with certain sounds cut out and see how much we can still understand. Depending on the material used we can go on understanding quite well, even if we are not able to hear every sound or every word, but then we are using our knowledge of language to help us fill in the gaps.

Listening practice is partly this: it is a means of training recognition of distorted sound; it is also practice in making sense of incomplete sentences; and it is practice in using listening in conjunction with lipreading for the best possible comprehension.

Speech Perception
Normal hearing people never need to think about the characteristics of the sounds they hear so easily. Neither is it imperative for the deafened to learn or go deeply into the

physics of sound, but people are interested to know something of what they actually can and cannot pick out from a sentence as it enables them to feel less foolish about the mistakes they are likely to make. If a listener is to distinguish between two sounds, for example the consonants s and sh, then he must be able to discriminate between a peaking of energy around 7,000 cycles, which characterizes the former, and a peaking of around 5,000 cycles, which is more typical of the latter. If it can be shown that, from his audiogram, he is unable to receive one of these frequencies then he has a clearer picture of the sounds to which he is actually deaf.

There are other features as well. It has already been noted that the consonant sounds may be divided into two broad classes — voiced and unvoiced. Since all consonant sounds involve the interruption or the constriction of the breath stream, they are all characterized by some kind of noise. However, the voiced consonants contain both this noise plus the complex tone of the vocal cords, so are more likely to be received than the unvoiced consonants. Other speech sounds can be identified by the way in which they evolve and also a time element — unvoiced plosives such as p, have a relatively abrupt start and they last only a short time. Unvoiced fricative consonants, such as f, on the other hand, have gradual onsets and last for relatively longer times. Of course, we do not deal with only one clue or feature of a sound in everyday listening, but such distinctions help us to realize that words and phrases reach our ears in patterns of sound and the ability to recognize patterns depends on learning.

Thus for good speech perception we require sensitivity to sound, discrimination of the sounds received, and recognition of sound patterns, plus the memory of our vocabulary and the structural aspects of our language. The basic notion of auditory perception is the ability to discriminate melodic features, which allow the listener to identify intonation patterns of the fundamental frequency of the voice. Such patterns are probably recognized very early by young children even before they begin to differentiate the speech sounds themselves. The implications of stress, rhythm and intonation are apparent in the following:

We usually leave here at four.
We *usually* leave here at four (but today we're leaving at a different time).
We usually leave at four (*they* go at another time).
We usually *leave* at four (not arrive).
We usually leave at *four*? (What are you talking about you fool?)

Even just two words can be said in various tones.

We are. (A plain statement.)
We *are*? (Are you sure?)
We are. (Whatever they might be doing.)
We *are*!!! (And that's an order!)

Stress may be *word* stress, which serves to distinguish between two meanings or uses of a word, or *sentence* stress, as just shown, to indicate the most important words in a phrase or sentence. The following are some examples of word stress:

We say the *im*ports and *ex*ports of the country; but the country im*ports* wheat and ex*ports* coal.
We talk of the Sunday *supp*lement; but a father supple*ments* his son's allowance.
He was an Au*gust* monarch, but we go on holiday in *Au*gust.

In auditory training it is better to start with sentence stress to catch the gross meaning of the message. Any finer analysis is not possible until the client is competent at this level.

Listening Practice
Listening practice is even more tiring than lipreading practice. In the latter we are encouraging a quick mental response; in the former we are trying to teach recognition of a new sound or sounds, as well as asking a client to distinguish similar melodic patterns. To concentrate on sound to this extent is very very tiring. Therefore such practice should be limited, in the early days, to a fifteen minute period, or even less if the client finds it exhausting, which means that progress may well be slow. On the other hand, if a few minutes of sound drill is given at each session,

followed by a connected piece based on the client's loss, then the concentration span is soon extended.

A typical lesson might be as follows. Clients seldom have only one listening problem, but the start of a session could be drill on one of the distortions. Let us say that there is confusion between the long and short vowels:

ee as in seat and i as in sit.

Then initial drill, first hearing the words repeated several times, then endeavouring to repeat one of the pairs said:

Drill

pitch	sin	whip	bit	hid
peach	seen	weep	beat	heed

The client ís not looking at the speaker, therefore he must be asked to look down, or to the side wall or at the written words put before him.

Used in sentences:

Which one am I using? The little boy — beat his sister.
                                         — bit his sister.

This exercise is to enable the listener to pick out the sound correctly in connected speech, when either word would make sense. Care should be taken not to stress the alternative words in an unnatural manner, that is, do not emphasize.

After the drill, a useful exercise can be illustrated with a short tape. For example the following, with the client watching as well as listening:

It's the usual weekend in the Jones household. Mrs Jones is in her kitchen. What do you think she's doing? (Sound of mixer or coffee grinder on tape.) Her daughter is sulking because she has been given a chore to do in the lounge. What do you think she's doing? (Sound of Hoover.) The husband is out in the garden. What do you think he's doing? (Sound of lawn mower or hedge clippers.) The eldest son is up in his bedroom. What do you think he's doing? (Sound of guitar or radio.) The other two boys are downstairs. What do you think this one is doing? (Sound of telephone dialling.) The other one is getting ready to go out with his girlfriend. What do you think he's doing? (Sound of shoe brushing or shaver.)

A more advanced example of this practice on

environmental sounds is as follows:

Miss Edwards had an exciting evening last night. Her boyfriend called for her at (sound of seven strikes from a clock). He asked her to meet him on the corner and he would pick her up in his (sound of car). Miss Edwards went out early. As she stood waiting she heard the sound of (crashing glass — broken window) and a man dashed round the corner. She heard a voice shouting (Stop him! Stop him!) and a shopkeeper came running, followed by (a barking dog). Suddenly she heard (a police whistle) and a policeman appeared at the other end of the street. The thief panicked and ran out into the road, just escaping a (lorry). It was all over in a few minutes. Miss Edwards heard (car hooter) and her boyfriend arrived. She was able to tell him the story as they drove away.

Similar pieces are useful to maintain a memory of the everyday sounds about us.

Spondee words are usually given during a speech audiometry test, but they are useful as practice material afterwards. These are words of two syllables in which each syllable can be used as a word on its own, for example — hothouse, ear-drum, sidewalk, horseshoe, headlight, daybreak, sunset, birthday, pancake. They may be used to listen to each portion separately, then as a complete word, and then picked out from a sentence.

Words which sound alike, although the spelling may be different, can be used to show that there is usually some other little word in the sentence which must be listened for in order to distinguish similar sentences. For example:

I think I'll buy four now.　The lipreading shape might
I think I'll pay for it now.　be similar but, when listen-
　　　　　　　　　　　　　　ing, there is a rhythm
　　　　　　　　　　　　　　change.

I can't afford the fare/I can't afford to go to the fair.

He bored a hole for the picture/he pored over the picture/he poured from the pitcher.

My hat blew off while shopping/my blue hat will do for shopping.

I wonder what scent she uses/I wonder what he sent you.

After some practice it may be possible to use even more

similar sentences, for example:

There is a rumour about.

    — a roamer about.

    — a rover about.

There is a fault below the house/there is a vault below the house.

He came in late/he came in laden.

What a chain of events/what a change of events.

The strain is terrible/the terrain is terrible/the train is terrible.

All these require very good powers of listening and are based on the sounds needed by individuals.

It is no great effort to make cards showing six colloquial sentences that have some common phrases repeated. The listener must wait until the end of each sentence to be sure of picking out or pointing to the correct one. For example:

Did you get soaked last night?

Did you get the storm at the weekend?

Wasn't it a terrible weekend!

Wasn't it a beautiful day yesterday!

Isn't the weather shocking!

Isn't it a shocking day!

Many auditory training manuals give lists and lists of words to be drilled and sentences with alternative endings, but if clients are to remain interested in listening I feel more varied material is necessary. As with lipreading, the mind plays a great part in deciphering aural signals and material should be presented which recognizes this factor. One way is to use a client's difficulty to compose some useful practice. If the deafened person has a problem recognizing the glottal stop, for instance, and has trouble with words such as little, bottle, kettle, settle, then something on the following lines could be composed:

I'm going to describe five bottles to you. You repeat what you think I say.

The first is a milk bottle.

The second is a beer bottle.

The third is a scent bottle. (Try perfume if scent is not recognized at all.)

The fourth is a bottle of tomato sauce.

The fifth is a bottle of aspirins.

The bottle of milk has a cap of silver foil. (Try gold if there is high frequency loss.)
The beer bottle has a metal cap.
The scent bottle has a glass stopper.
The bottle of tomato sauce has a screw top.
The bottle of aspirins has a safety top.

Let me tell you what I do when the bottles are empty.
I put out the milk bottle for the milkman.
I take the beer bottle back to the off-licence.
I put the scent bottle in a drawer amongst my clothes.
I throw the sauce bottle into the rubbish bin.
I take the aspirin bottle back to the chemist.
In this way there is much repetition of and listening for the word 'bottle'.

Number work can be done in several ways — such as conversational drill in which the listener picks out and repeats the number he hears:
My train was twelve minutes late.
It takes me two hours to get here.
I shall be fifty-three in March.
There were about 150 at the meeting.
My new flat has five rooms, with a lounge twenty feet long.
The flat is on the fifth floor.

It is helpful to keep material to a theme, at least in the early stages of training. For example, ask the listener to pick out the profession or job that he hears in these sentences.
I must go to see my solicitor.
My daughter wants to be a nurse.
I have a brother who works in advertising.
Our dustmen call on Thursdays.
I'm looking for a domestic help.
Did you go to a tailor for that suit?
Our bus conductor was so rude this morning.
I must make an appointment to see an optician.

Introducing *background noise* is something which listeners hate initially but find, with practice, they can learn to ignore. The wireless operator has to train his ear to focus on a particular callsign and pick this out from a number of other Morse signals going out on the air. This seems an impossibility at first but, with training, the operator finds no difficulty in excluding those signals he doesn't want. Since deafened people complain that one of the worst ordeals is to sit in noisy restaurants, learning to concentrate through or above unwanted noise can be worthwhile. To start, a tape of café conversation can be played at low volume while the teacher recites a few numbers. Once these have become easy to repeat back the background volume can be increased and everyday sentences tried. It is another means of focussing attention and developing powers of listening.

Sound Waves

Sound waves do peculiar things. They reflect from hard surfaces and they can also reflect at angles. Because of this we get unusual effects, such as whispering galleries like the one in St. Paul's Cathedral, where the sound seems to creep round the walls so that a soft voice is still audible at astonishing distances. Sometimes sitting in front of large window surfaces, or in the angle formed by two walls with a hard surface, can increase the intensity of sound for a person who is hard of hearing, but more often than not the poor absorption power of surfaces make hearing more difficult. Hard plaster walls and glazed tile surfaces have very poor powers of absorption so that sound waves bounce back from these surfaces and the sound echoes are sent back, albeit in weaker form, to the receiver of the hearing aid. Too great a reverberation interferes seriously with the understanding of speech, as the listener is forced to rely on context to understand syllables which have been distorted by overlapping waves. Therefore someone who is hard of hearing will hear very much better in a room which has been acoustically treated with tiles with holes or acoustic felts, and it is helpful in homes to have carpet with felt underpads on the floor, and heavy curtains with folds at window areas, to prevent reverberation. However, all these materials are absorbing sound as well as preventing echo so the person who is hard of hearing needs to be quite close to the speaker in order to understand.

The person with a conductive type of deafness is even more at a disadvantage in a room with very high sound absorption than the person with a nerve type of deafness. This is because the conductively-deaf person needs a relatively higher volume of sound for the same degree of hearing loss. He would be better in a home furnished with metallic furniture, glass-topped tables and wood floors.

Another effect of sound absorption is felt in the open air. Many people with impaired hearing will say that they feel lost at an outdoor party or picnic, and this is because sound in the open air is simply dispersed without anything to deflect or reflect it.

Sound travels in waves at a rate of 760 miles an hour. These waves cause changes of pressure in the ear and these changes alternate between increases and decreases of pressure. One of these double vibrations performs one cycle, and the number of cycles per second made by any sound is called its frequency. The human ear is unable to perceive sound waves as sound until these vibrations reach 20 cycles per second, so our ears start to hear the lowest tone at 20 cycles a second and the sensation of sound, to human ears, disappears at about 20,000 cycles.

Without doubt the ear is a miracle of reception, able to deal with a barrage of varying sounds and noises throughout life, never resting and, seldom still. There is, we are told, a fluid in our inner ear that appears to have the same consistency as sea water, so perhaps it was evolved under water and the drum prevented the sea getting in. However, it is limited in the volume of noise it can stand without suffering damage.

The Volume of Sound
Intensity of sound, or loudness, is measured in decibels. This is a convenient measure because one decibel, very roughly, is equal to the least difference in loudness which is perceptible to the human ear. The noise in a bedroom at night would be between 20–30 decibels; a living-room in a suburban area between 40–50 decibels; conversational speech would be between 60–70 decibels; average traffic on a street corner 70–80; a pop group might approximate 110 decibels; a loud car horn 120; a pneumatic drill 130 — and now we are on the threshold of pain. Obviously our ears are accepting different intensities of sound all and every day, but if we are in too intense a noise for a long period then our ear does protest and, although it may recover, it does not fully return to its previous acuity. This

is the danger that people are exposed to if they work in very noisy industrial surroundings, or if they are exposed to loud music for long periods of time. It does not cause immediate deafness but is an insidious loss that can build up to severity with time.

The statement 'People are beginning to mumble' is usually brought forward as a sign that deafness is encroaching. On the other hand it is rather horrifying to read a table of the volume of sound used by speakers. Research was carried out by an American, E.H. Colpitts, the results of which have been published in the Bell System Technical Journal. He related the ratio of power of individual speakers' voices to the average power of speech. He took as his yardstick the following accepted table:

Loud speech is about 10 decibels higher than the norm (accepted as 50/60 decibels);
Very loud speech is about 20 decibels higher;
Faint speech is about 10 decibels weaker than the norm;
Very faint speech is about 20 decibels weaker;
A whisper is 10 decibels below very faint.

From this he deduced the following:
7 per cent of all speakers speak with only $\frac{1}{16}$ the power of the average voice;
9 per cent speak with only $\frac{1}{16}$ to $\frac{1}{8}$ the power;
14 per cent speak with only $\frac{1}{8}$ to $\frac{1}{4}$ the power;
18 per cent speak with only $\frac{1}{4}$ to $\frac{1}{2}$ the power;
If we add the percentages so far then we see that 48 per cent of those tested spoke with half or less the power of the average voice.

He completes his table:
22 per cent of speakers used between $\frac{1}{2}$ to 1 normal power;
17 per cent used normal or twice the power;
9 per cent used twice or four times the power;
Therefore 4 per cent must have had very powerful voices with over 4 times the power.

Men's voices have a lower pitch and more power. Women's pitch is about an octave higher — middle C on the piano. However, these are merely the carrier waves produced by the larynx; the complex speech sounds which differentiate our vowels and consonants are from 2–4 octaves higher. So the deafened person must expect many of the people he meets to have quiet, non-carrying voices.

Another cause of the weakening of sound intensity is distance from the source or the speaker. Every person with a hearing loss should know that the relationship between sound intensity and distance follows the inverse square law. This means that sound does not get fainter, on a 1-to-1 or 2-to-2 basis as the distance increases. Instead it varies inversely as the square of the distance from the source. Simply, it means that if you are standing in the open air listening to somebody speaking at close range, let us say a distance of *two* feet, and the speaker moves away to a distance of *four* feet, his voice is not one-half as loud as it was but *one-fourth* as loud. If he continues to move further away to a distance of *eight* feet his voice is not one-fourth as loud but *one-sixteenth*. If he goes off to a distance of *sixteen* feet his voice will then become only one-*sixty-fourth* as loud. Therefore, the person who is hard of hearing has to learn to make a concerted effort to be within his own conversational range — he has to discover for himself the approximate range he must be in for normal conversational speech.

This law applies with full force only outdoors, or in rooms that are fairly sound absorbent and non-reflective. In many rooms and closed areas, the sound cannot escape easily so that the sound waves tend to be bounced back and forth. If the bounce-back effect of untreated rooms is too great there is considerable speech confusion and loss of intelligibility.

Today the science of acoustics is well-recognized and no major public building would be constructed without careful planning of the acoustic conditions. Acoustic scientists work constantly to reduce noise in cars, aeroplanes and home appliances; while acoustic physicists strive to improve the sound reproduction of television, radio, public address systems, and other recording equipment. For the hard of hearing today are faced with a vastly different situation than the hard of hearing of fifty years ago. The world in which they live is far noisier; it is more mechanized; and for much of the time they are listening to sound and voices which have been electrically recorded and transmitted and amplified. It would pay them to learn a little about acoustics if they are to manage more easily in this modern electronic age.

Auditory training would seem to be dependent on the degree of loss; that is, it would be expected that a person with a *slight* loss of hearing would more easily distinguish sounds, both environmental and speech. In practice this is not always so. Sometimes a person with a *severe* loss will, with training and motivation, learn to 'listen' so hard and put together aural clues that he is able to use the telephone and appear far less deaf than his pure tone result would indicate.

The deaf face the difficulty of belonging to a minority group living in a world of hearing people. Their own attitude to their deafness may depend on the feelings they had about deaf people before they suffered their own loss. A person's self-esteem is often affected and this, in turn, either leads him to expect too much from a rehabilitation course, or his lack of esteem does not allow him to achieve all he could. Thus it is not possible to gauge an individual's probability of success merely by reading his hearing chart or scoring a speech audiometry test. Much will depend on a training course, which will take the factor of self-esteem into consideration because of its dominant influence on the adjustment process and future achievement.

It is, therefore, important in the early stages of diagnosis and issuing of the aid that the deafened person is made fully aware of what it is possible for him still to hear, of how to get the best possible performance from any device he is issued with, and of the need to use his residual hearing to the full. Remember that deduction of the sound source is not enough; there must be interpretation of the sound if hearing is to be relevant. Certainly the purely biological function is important but it is the highly developed sophisticated use of sound as communication which matters in society.

4

LIPREADING

Take care of the sense, and the sounds will take care of themselves.

The Duchess in *Alice in Wonderland*.

What is Lipreading?

Lipreading certainly cannot be exactly what the name indicates. If lips only were read, then no sensible language would result from merely deciphering the visible movements. It has been termed 'an art'; others call it a skill; yet others endeavour to prove that it cannot be taught as a subject.

Whatever opinion one favours, there are certain truths that cannot be gainsaid, despite the fact that it is still not known quite what lipreaders do when they understand an aural language (i.e. received by the ear) by using a visual method. A public misconception is that when a deafened person says 'I am a lipreader' all he has to do is to watch the speaker and complete comprehension is possible. It is a far more complicated matter than this. To start with, no two lipreaders are similarly placed: their hearing loss is probably quite different, they may or may not be able to use an aid, their sight may vary, the speaker they face may be clear, or mumble, or speak too fast, or be a foreigner. All these are factors upon which 'ease of lipreading' must be based.

Who Can Lipread?

Research shows, and my own experience of experimenting with a hearing audience bears out, the fact that we all can lipread to varying degrees. A hearing audience will quickly lipread numbers, a simple story, a few remarks — making the same mistakes as would a deaf audience. There are the same wide variations in skill — one person seemingly able to lipread everything said, and others finding the going hard, and yet others giving up along the way. What is not realized is that it may be no great effort to lipread a few numbers, or follow a short story, but to keep this up from the time you wake until bedtime is a very different matter. A lipreader not only has to keep 'with' speakers and maintain utter concentration, but to cope with a gallery of faces and mouths, wide lips, thin lips, protruding teeth, invisible tongues, cavernous mouths, immovable lips, bearded chins, wagging heads — all manner of human physiognomy that can make lipreading more difficult.

We all, unconsciously perhaps, experience the need to lipread. If we are in a noisy situation, where the sound level of the noise is greater than that of the human voice, then we must look at the speaker in order to understand him. Deaf people themselves often forget or fail to realize that hearing people cannot listen to a number of voices at once. A common remark from a deafened adult is, 'I find I cannot hear in a room full of people'. I find myself, although I possess very good hearing, that I am in the same position where there is background music and a hubbub of speech; I have to look at the person speaking to me and really concentrate on what he is trying to tell me. Our ears do not have such a wide receiving range that they can pick up all frequencies or, more particularly, our speech range is so limited that it doesn't take very much loud extraneous noise to drown a speaking voice. If this were not so I should have no need of phrases that I use regularly such as, 'What did you say?' 'I didn't get that,' and 'I beg your pardon'.

I could, no doubt, train my ears to work a little harder and, as radio operators do in their work, learn to pick out signals I need from others round about. But since I probably have a good clue as to subject matter, and can make sense from a few operative words, then I rely on hearing enough to manage very well in most situations. However, without hearing the operative words there would be many occasions when I might misunderstand, or just not know what is going on. It is this for which the deafened person is finding a substitute, by honing his visual ability — learning to use clues consciously so that the brain is receiving some signal to decipher.

A normal adult is sending his brain a signal from his hearing apparatus, plus one from his eyes, the combination of which enables his mental ability to comprehend speech. With one signal missing or impaired, the brain has less upon which to work and, as will be seen from later examples, confusion is likely to arise from the structure of our language. On the other hand, we do have a very rich language; it is always possible to find an alternative, perhaps a more lipreadable word or turn of phrase, and this is one way in which the public could relieve frustration and embarrassment for the hard of hearing — by seeking another way of saying something rather than continuing to repeat the original phrase.

Since there has always been deafness, it would seem that there have always been people who have had to lipread. Lipreading has been formally taught for centuries and before that must have been learned informally ever since man has used speech to communicate. There are many people now who lipread well who have never had formal training, yet manage to do so because of their natural ability to transpose shapes into meaning. But with the increased awareness of the problem of deafness, and the attempts at rehabilitation, formal training is now becoming available to many more people.

Lipreading Past and Present
We know that lipreading was practised as early as the sixteenth century, and taught by the Spaniard Ponce de Leon, but before this were the dark ages of the deaf, which were a chaos of tragedy and ignorance.

Towards the end of the fifteenth century, when the Renaissance was beginning to extend its influence and inspire individuals with the idea of teaching the deaf, we find reports of deaf individuals being taught to speak and understand others. There are mentions of deaf painters, and poets also, who were accepted as intelligent beings and allowed to use their talents to lead a full life. But it was from Spain that the first teacher of the deaf came. Pedro Ponce de Leon was a monk, who had for his pupils deaf and dumb youths who were the sons of great lords but whose estates they forfeited because of their handicap. He taught them to speak, read, write and pray and his greatest success was with two deaf brothers whom he taught to speak and lipread.

At the start of the seventeenth century a number of books were published concerning the deaf and teachers in different parts of Europe began to evolve various methods of instruction. Another Spaniard, Juan Bonet, became teacher to a noble family where deafness was hereditary and he published a book explaining his methods of teaching speech, which are surprisingly modern, simple and practical. But on the subject of lipreading he is not so modern. He thought that lipreading should not be taught and that no system could be devised to teach this.

In England a number of persons began to show interest in the deaf. In the past, monks of silent orders had become skilled in the use of signs and some of them also practised lipreading. A man named John Bulwer wrote a philosophical book quoting this, and the fact that even schoolboys had learned to read lips in school when they were prevented from speaking. Also, one assumes that prisoners everywhere would have tried to make some form of contact with each other, using lip movements.

Heinicke in Germany was the great teacher of the deaf who was convinced of the need for the deaf to communicate normally. This is shown in his repeated insistence that clear thought is possible only by speech and, therefore, that the deaf ought to be taught to speak and understand the speech of others from the motion of the lips. In this country the Braidwood family kept this oral method alive and it is due to these methods of teaching deaf children how to lipread that the methods for teaching adults have evolved.

Teachers of the Deaf in America met as a convention for the first time in 1850 in New York. Their official organ was *The American Annals of the Deaf and Dumb* and through its pages teachers recorded their experiences in teaching lipreading — experiences which still hold good today. The little group of oral teachers had been taught the use of 'visible speech' by Alexander Graham Bell, whose wife and sister both suffered deafness. There are many accounts and letters from successful lipreaders, and others from teachers of lipreading, describing their methods. Many reveal that the old preoccupation with positions of speech still dominated teaching at this time, but much of this was contradicted by the lipreaders themselves who wrote of their own attainments and experiences.

The most outstanding paper was that from Mrs Alexander Graham Bell, which was so far ahead of its time that it may still be read today as a modern exposition of lipreading. Mrs Bell stressed the necessity of being able to read rapid speech and insisted that the synthetic method of practice was more useful than the previous stress with positions. She pointed out that, because of the large number of words that are alike to the eye, the art of reading speech depends on grasping the meaning as a whole rather than trying to decipher single words. The mind is then trained from the beginning to fill in the blanks and to make an instant guess at what is being said. She found this the best method for herself and said that anyone with a quick, bright mind and a good knowledge of language could develop into a fair speech reader. Her exposition did not immediately change the teaching of lipreading, but gradually teaching methods were simplified and became less theory and more practice. The work of lipreading became more impressive and its acquisition was regarded more as a matter of study than sheer accident.

The lipreading teachers of the past were usually working on an individual basis, teaching deaf children during the day and taking a deaf adult after school hours. One teacher wrote a little pamphlet called, 'Speech Reading; a Guide for Self-Instruction where trained teachers are not available', which was illustrated with pictures of the speech positions. The pupil was told to watch himself in a mirror and helpful sentences were given to practise.

Most of the teachers who were working in America at this time, using Professor Bell's *Principles of Speech and Dictionary of Sounds* went about the work on the theory that facility in lipreading just grew. From what we read of reports of Miss Hamilton, a teacher who was able to instruct an adult in the speech not only of Americans but also foreigners after only twelve weeks, it appears that teaching was done without voice. One man said that when he lipread, his knowledge of the language was so natural that he had to place his hand on the teacher's back to assure himself that she was actually not using her voice.

It is interesting to learn that as early as 1884 a convention was asked why teachers of lipreading received no specific training, as did teachers of speech, because it was not until 1970 that any such training scheme was permanently planned in this country. A start had been made after the Second World War by the RNID, who trained a small number of teachers to deal with the problem of ex-servicemen deafened as a result of their war experiences, but this proved only a temporary measure.

In 1884 some opinions were very advanced for the time. A Miss Keeler said that she applied one of Pestalozzi's principles to her teaching of lipreading, i.e. she proceeded from the obvious to the obscure, devoting the first part of her lessons to drills on sounds and sentences, and then using the last part for dictation of connected language and conversation.

Perhaps the person who has had the most original ideas in the field of lipreading was Edward Nitchie. He became very deaf whilst in his teens but managed to finish his studies at the side of hearing boys. He had difficulty in finding work but eventually secured an editorial post with the Church Council. He had never heard of lipreading at this time but when a friend suggested he join a class he enrolled, only to find that, because he had a logical, analytical type of mind, it was not easy. Nitchie realized the possibilities of lipreading, and wanted to teach it himself, and when he was only 26 he opened a studio in New York where he gave courses to children who were hard of hearing. However, he soon had so many applications from adults that he left the school side of the work and devoted himself to developing his method of lipreading instruction. Nitchie's first book showed an analytical approach and still resembled methods used with the born deaf. Later he abandoned the rather illogical exercises and each book showed a marked progress in dealing with the synthetic grasp of mental processes.

During this century we have had the benefit of improvements in hearing aids and research into learning factors, with special reference to adult learning and the work being done on speech recognition. Yet we still cannot better the teaching skills of these pioneers who recognized the need for analysis as well as synthesis to practise lipreading and who had to devise all their own material for lessons.

So what makes a good lipreader, what is lipreading and why is it not possible for everyone to attain the highest standard?

I have found that most clients come with too high an expectation of what is possible. They have read of deaf people able to carry on their work, often in highly professional jobs, because of their ability to lipread, and assume that a short course of instruction will work a miracle for them. They do not stop to consider that from the thousands of musicians able to play a violin, few reach the standard of Yehudi Menuhin, or that of all the tens of thousands of small boys kicking a football, few will attain the skill of a George Best. Few lipreaders become real champions but even a little aptitude helps and clients require much encouragement in the early stages, and often reminders as to whether, if they were learning to play the piano, they would give up after a few weeks if they were not invited to play at the Festival Hall! As with other enthusiasms, the first flush soon wears off. Preliminary classes are easy, since a good teacher would make them so, but after comes the dull hard slog with perhaps no visible progress and this is when a client is more likely to continue if only he has the support of a teacher or spouse to keep him going.

Losing some hearing has no counterpart with losing some sight. The eyes can be instantly corrected after testing and life continues normally; a loss of hearing denotes being cut off from much that was possible before. In fact, those becoming totally deaf to speech must put aside the desire for sounds, for hearing the human voice, and enjoying music. Their answer is to use their lipreading to the utmost of their ability, realizing its limitations and when it breaks down, as it will quite often, reviewing the situation with humour rather than despair. Leisure time has to be filled with activities which do not depend on sound.

Some Common Questions
Is there an age limit, or am I too old to learn? The answer is No.

If I wear a hearing aid, and hear well with it do I need lipreading? Yes, because no hearing aid is infallible; most hearing loss is progressive so that lipreading is a good insurance against future loss.

Who is the best lipreader? Must you be young, old, brainy? A natural lipreader is the best, but everyone can reach some rung of the ladder and find the skill useful.

What makes a good lipreader? Concentration and agility of mind are probably the most important factors, although personality plays a large part in overcoming problems.

How long will it take me to learn? Learning never finishes; it is something you will be doing for the rest of your life. Lipreading is an art and, as such, has to be continually practised. Some people progress faster than others, as in any art.

How can I tell that I am lipreading if I can hear with a hearing aid? Probably when someone covers their mouth and you find you can't hear and you get annoyed about this, or when you find you can't hear so well in the dark or a noisy place.

The Attitude of Others

Of course, the attitude of hearing people is often thoughtless, sometimes to the point of mental cruelty. This may be due to their ignorance, or lack of imagination, or unwillingness to make any effort. Most deaf people will recognize the following common instances:

A deaf person is invited to a small party of friends, one group may be talking about one subject, often leaning over to talk to each other, another group discuss something else, and the deaf person is left out. Then lipreading cannot help much without a willing helper.

There is unfortunately the common incident of the deaf person asking, 'What's the joke?' having seen a general burst of laughter, and being told 'Oh, it's not worth repeating,' or 'It's nothing much'.

There can even be the unkind, 'It's no good talking to you — you never hear,' or, even worse, to have someone ask over your head, 'Does he take sugar?'

'Oh you heard that — you can hear when you want to,' is the most difficult to blame, since the speaker cannot be expected to know that some sentences *will* be heard and others not, depending on the visibility of the words used.

These are but a few of many such everyday incidents, none of which will help to relieve the burden of the affliction.

But lipreading is more than a crutch to enable some communication to continue. It can be a renewal of interest in tackling an interesting skill; it can be something to be proud of doing when you achieve some ability, and should give pleasure when done well.

What Makes a Good Lipreader?

What have the researchers found out? They say that lipreading is thought to be easier for people with good *visual perception*; good *speed* of perception and general *visual proficiency*. Obviously good eyesight is important and lipreaders should have this checked regularly. Also, an observant person is likely to gain more facial clues; while good peripheral vision enables the lipreader to absorb other information while still focusing on the mouth of the speaker.

Incidental to this point, I think it is helpful for a client to be shown simple exercises that will relieve eye strain. Beginners concentrate so hard that they are inclined to over-stare and are afraid to move the head, so that a few relaxing movements ease strain and fatigue. As a further point on the business of concentration, I remember reading one report on eye movement which stressed the fact that everyone has a different rate of blinking the eyes, and that perhaps a slow lipreader was someone who blinked too much and so missed mouth movements while his eyes were momentarily shut. A week or two later I read yet another report which stated the opposite — that a rapid 'blinker' might be a better lipreader because his quick movements tied up with rapid mental processes. So *that* one is obviously unproven.

The second important point is to have a good *synthetic ability*, which means the ability to make an intelligent guess at missing language — to be able to fill in missing details and combine fragments into a meaningful whole. I do think that the ability to draw conclusions is very important, partly on the level of filling in missing shapes and partly at the higher level of supplying missing words. To organize and group

ᐧ the words which have been perceived into a tentative idea is the basis of lipreading ability. For those with a more analytical mind this is often a difficult hurdle — they worry at missing a word, want or expect to see every shape, and consequently lose the framework of the general idea.

Good *flexibility* is said to be important, which means being able to free the mind of a concept which is incorrect and revise the original conclusion. As many sounds are homophenous, i.e. they look the same because they are made by using the same mouth movements, this means that many words will also make similar shapes. We all know that their and there, four, for, and fore, rows, rose and roes, have like sounds and, to the lipreader, present like shapes. But the lipreader has additional homophenous words and phrases, due to his inability to hear any difference between voiced and unvoiced sound, or to see any difference in the rhythms of speech. An example would be where the sounds made by p, b, and m would be clear enough to a hearing person but make the same shape to someone with a hearing loss, which would result in the words batch, match, and patch looking alike. This has the same effect in other positioning of the letters, so that rim, rib, and rip would present a similar problem. Such similar combinations as, 'You're in my light,' 'You're in a plight,' and 'You're impolite,' would also require careful deciphering.

It is this particular problem which makes class attendance worthwhile. If a client understands this matter of homophenes and learns the 'family' sounds, he is less likely to think himself stupid if a mistake is made, and is more able to be flexible enough to make a quick mental change and choose a message which is meaningful and appropriate.

Social and situational awareness
This is the necessity for continuing to mix with people, watch faces, lips, body movements, and endeavour to sum up a situation in order to be aware of language that is likely to be used at that time, or with those people, or in that place.

Training in lipreading
There has been controversy over the question whether lipreading *can* be taught. In my experience, children born

deaf *have* to be taught in order to survive, so I cannot doubt that adults may also learn. The question may have arisen because most people who attend classes have already learned to lipread to some degree; in fact they may well have reached their capacity, since many do not start a class until they have been deaf for several years. Such people have suffered a progressive loss which has been so gradual that they have taught themselves to watch people when the speaker has a quiet voice, so that when they do come to a class, either because they have lost the final remnant of speech sounds and feel 'very deaf', or because it has been suggested that they attend when they have visited an audiology centre for a new aid, they are not beginners. Although these people gain other benefits from classes they may not improve their ability.

It has been my experience that many need to be put into an advanced group of lipreaders immediately, since their ability is already good. Only the relatively few, who are made suddenly deaf from trauma or through illness, can be said to be starting from scratch. I think it is important that they receive individual help and intensive practice during the first weeks of attendance as, because they have not had time to absorb the shock of not hearing sound, many are intensely bothered by tinnitus, and counselling and support are essential.

I have also found that even very good lipreaders can be made better — speed can be increased, language structures practised, and work given for mental stimulation. Although a good teacher wishes to lose a pupil as soon as possible when he is ready to cope outside classroom walls, even the best lipreaders like to return at intervals for a short refresher course to maintain their skill at a high level.

Emotional attitudes
Since our emotions affect our ability to relax, our motivation, our fear of failure, our willingness to make a fool of ourselves, our willingness to 'have a go', and our ability to concentrate and to persevere, lipreaders will react in the same way as learners of other skills. How many ardent would-be potters sign on for evening classes, or hopeful linguists for language classes, and never stay the course? Lipreaders are not quite in the same position. They

may have been told that they *must* come to a class because they will be deafer in later life and lipreading would be a form of insurance; they may have been forced to attend through family pressure or fear of losing employment — attitudes which are not conducive to ease of learning.

It is, therefore, very important initially to give everyone a realistic goal. They must know and have it often repeated that, despite any skill they may attain, there will always be situations in which lipreading is impossible, that it is limited by distance and by eyesight, that it is almost entirely dependent on being fed a possible lipreadable pattern, and that it may well be necessary, for a peaceful life, to choose friends and activities as they relate to the possibilities of lipreading. Being deaf *does* curtail activities; it *does* limit social intercourse; it *is* tiring, frustrating and depressing; and it is the devil to live with. But with the courage to attempt lipreading, and the support of other deaf class members and a tutor, there is some lightening of the way and personal satisfaction that you are doing something to alleviate the disability rather than wallow in utter misery.

Some General Points

Let us then, before studying the intricacies of lipreading, list some general points to remember:

1. *Acknowledge your hearing impairment.* (This is not the easiest thing to do, it may be a long time before you accept that speakers are not mumbling, it is your hearing that is deteriorating). If you think you are not hearing normally, or are worried in any way, make an appointment to see your doctor who will arrange for you to have a hearing test.

2. *Try not to hide it or be ashamed of it.* Again, this is something that is easier to say than to carry out. I do understand that the deaf would rather wear the small post-aural aid that is invisible when under the hair, but this also hides the fact of their handicap. I well remember the mother of a small deaf boy who regularly sent him to school with his hearing aid, the body-worn variety, pushed down into the back pocket of his trousers. Since she made no attempt also to hide the spectacles he was wearing, it was sad that she should associate his not hearing with some

shame, whereas a loss of sight appeared acceptable. When asked, her reply was that if people saw the boy was deaf, they would think he was daft. My point was that he would certainly be daft if she left it in his trousers since the microphone on the aid was then as far away from a speaker's voice as it was possible to be, and he wouldn't understand a word.

There still does appear to be some hangover from the past, when the born deaf were literally dumb because no attempts were made to teach them to speak and most would appear rather stupid and slow because of their lack of understanding. Also, life was shorter and many people died in their forties before a progressive deafness made much impact. But now, with the ever-increasing number of sufferers, one would trust that the feeling of any shame would not be countenanced.

It is most important to have a positive attitude towards any disability in order to take useful measures to deal with it successfully.

3. *Use a hearing aid* that is properly selected and seek professional help if it does not appear to be working properly.

4. *Position yourself* so that you can see the speaker's face clearly whenever possible.

5. *Maintain a sense of humour.* It isn't funny to be deaf, but many of the mis-readings will be and both you and the speaker will feel less tense if you are able to laugh at errors. Don't be ashamed to ask for a repeat but remember to wait until the speaker has finished. If you interrupt you may have missed a vital clue at the end of a sentence.

6. *Don't monopolize a conversation.* This is a common failing with the deaf. Since lipreading is very tiring, and so many people are poor speakers, it is tempting to monopolize conversation in an attempt to avoid lipreading. But conversation is a two-way activity and your companions will become very annoyed if you don't let them get a word in edgeways or if you don't *try* to understand what they are saying.

7. *Keep up with the world.* Read the newspapers and

maintain a wide range of interests so that you know what people are likely to talk about from day to day. Keep building your lipreading vocabularly, especially colloquial expressions.

Don't be discouraged if you have bad days when lipreading seems impossible. The best lipreaders have 'off' days and they don't understand everything by lipreading alone.

8. *Educate your circle.* It will be mainly *your* responsibility to educate your family and friends. You can put people at ease by suggesting how they might help you — speaking clearly, changing words, giving you a clue. They may know you are deaf but they don't automatically know how to help. If you were blind it would be more obvious what help you needed, but until the public are made aware of the fleeting lip movements and the illusive structure of the language, you will need to tell them *what* they can do to help you to understand their speech.

If you find that your relations with normal-hearing people are not good, do not blame this on your lipreading. It might be something else about you, your appearance or your manner for instance, but it is just as likely to be the other person's attitude towards deafness that is at fault.

Above all, if you wish to be a lipreader who can be proud of his skill, then practise, practise, *practise!*

Lipreading Classes
Before I attempt to show that by teaching lipreading we are teaching language, where do you go for lipreading tuition and what is available? Unless you reside in a remote part of the country, then it is likely that there will be at least one class available where you could receive lipreading tuition. However, even in London and other major cities, it is unlikely that a class would be on your doorstep and fares and transport become additional headaches. There are still very few areas where you would have the choice of a morning, afternoon or evening class on every day of the week, or have the choice of a class graded to your abilities. But it is possible that a club for the hard of hearing is in your vicinity and most of these provide lipreading tuition and practice. A list of useful addresses will be given at the end of

the book (pages 234–6) if you wish to make enquiries about facilities in your area.

The advantages of joining a class of lipreaders are that you will find other deaf people possibly worse off than you, able to give you encouragement; you will have someone to measure progress by; and you will find companionship and be able to relax and exchange ideas. For others, individual help is essential, particularly for those who are true beginners because of sudden, total deafness, for those for whom English may not be their native tongue, for the experienced lipreader who feels time is wasted in class, or for those professionals requiring a specific vocabulary.

If there is no help available at all where you live then you need the help of a friend who will give you time to practise through conversation or the help of graded exercises. To help yourself, apart from lipreading, you can seek information about lights, clocks, telephones, and additional aids; you can train *observation* to help take the place of *hearing*; you can put glass in doors so that you can see someone is there; you can learn to laugh at yourself and your mistakes; and, very important, you can grow a thicker skin.

Lipreading and Language

The lipreader is required to forget the written pattern of the words he knows, that is, to him the spelling is no longer important. What *is* important is the sound the letters make, because from the sound he will receive the shape to watch. For example, we spell sugar s, u, g, a, r, but as the sound of s in this word is sh, then the lipreader is looking for the shape *sh*ugar. If you consider the word 'circus', and listen as you say it, you will note that the first c is sounded as s and the second as a k, which is how the lipreader must visualize it. Similarly with vowel sounds, the letters er represent the long vowel er as in fern, but the sound represents also the spellings *ir*, as in bird, *or*, as in worm, *ur*, as in fur, *ear*, as in earth, *yr*, as in myrhh.

However, if a word should end in er, as in water, the long vowel is not stressed in speech and the er is said as the neutral, e.g., 'My daught*a* will be 21 tomorrow'. To the lipreader the word one begins with the shape of w since we do not say on-ee, hence 'I wunce visited China'.

The letters ow represent the sound ow as in how, flowers, and shower. But should a word end in ow as in pillow, the final ow changes its sound so that we ask, 'Would you like the windo open?' And, to make learning more complicated, ow is not always representative of the same sound, as, for example, in such sentences as — the actor took a bow, but — the girl wore a bow in her hair. Or, with two examples in the same sentence, 'Don't those flowers look lovely in that bowl!'

Consonants are also interchangeable. To a lipreader, unable to hear voice, the letters f/v/ph make a similar shape. Transpose these into words and *few* will look like *view*, and *fillip* like *Phillip* so that a sentence such as, 'Phillip took a very fine photograph' would offer a lipreader some very good shapes but, as a beginner, some mental problems.

Language is designed for the ear and not the eye. We are dependent on hearing the pitch and tone of voice to know whether we have been asked a question or query; we decipher rapid speech by the rhythm of phrases and we never think about homophenous words because we hear sufficient clues to sort these out from meaning. Think of the anomolies, also the pleasure, of language: if you are knocked *down* you may be laid *up* for a time. People cut *down* trees and then they cut them *up*.

We have thousands and thousands of examples of the fun of language in word jokes: 'If you were invited out to dinner and saw only a beetroot on the table, what would you say?' That beet's all. 'What changed the dairyman's luck?' He found a whey (way) to make money.

We are amused by such word play because we do not have the task of first making sense of similar shapes before we can appreciate a nuance. Just try to imagine a lipreader coping with, 'And I wish that I knew what that new gnu knew!'

Perhaps a better description of lipreading would be the term 'speech reading' since we are asking the deaf to read colloquial language rather than the written form. In addition to this we are asking them to lipread a great deal of ungrammatical English, since our thoughts are usually expressed too quickly for us always to construct a correctly phrased sentence. I spent some time a few years ago taping conversations that I heard, mainly within the limits of a place of work, but also in different environments. At the time I was having grave doubts about the type of material which we, as teachers, were presenting to classes. Our lessons, however carefully planned, were from the written form in the main and I was of the opinion that most of the lesson time should be spent in practice on everyday language in situations that would be common to most of us. Here are a few of the examples I gathered:

'Did you get caught in the rain?'

'Not really — it wasn't bad enough to come in out of from.'

'I like her but I don't like her like I like Margaret.'

Two ladies arguing about a book one had lent to the other — 'Then why did you give it to me to read out of from for?'

'So I said to him, "Oh," and he said, "Oh, it's Oh is it?" and I said "Yes, it is Oh." '

There is very little, in any of these, for the lipreader to hinge his interpretation upon, and all are far removed from much of the material normally presented in class.

Words are mysteries that we live with from day to day. No one truly knows how language came into being, how man converted what must have been an animal cry into the complicated systems of articulated speech. Indeed we rarely think of the miracle of speech — how a thought in one person's mind can be transferred to the listener's mind, through a series of nervous impulses by organs of speech, and then received into the listener's ear, where the whole process goes into reverse so that the message may be accepted and understood. All of this happens in mere seconds of time. But it is possible only when two people are communicating in the same language — when we are 'on each other's wavelength' — so that, for ease of communication, a lipreader must have a good knowledge of his own tongue.

We don't know why there should be so many languages: does language really exist in the singular like music or are there only languages which must remain permanently foreign to each other, so long as they survive at all? It is not surprising that many people have yearned for linguistic simplification, for example, Esperanto, but if this had caught on its words would probably have immediately begun to develop complexities of meaning in order to cover the range of human thought. In more recent times it was supposed that computers would be able to simplify the transfer of word meaning from one language to another. But the pioneers quickly discovered that this is only feasible between scientific vocabularies in which each term has a set single meaning and the relationship between the terms can be reduced to a simple, syntactical pattern. It would need a wise machine to be able to recognize the relevant meaning of any ambiguous everyday word. For example, how would it distinguish between steps and stairs in English, and between the grammatical simple and continuous present as in I make/I am making?

It is easy to see in translation how a language is its own master. The slogan 'Come alive with Pepsi' was rendered too literally in the Taiwan market — in Chinese it read, 'Pepsi brings your ancestors back from the grave'. While in Japanese, 'Out of sight, Out of mind' becomes 'Invisible, insane'.

It is quite a disconcerting experience to be shown an exact transcript of a conversation in which you have taken part. The incoherence, the gaps, the hesitations, the habits of speech, and the repetitions are shocking to read and this is because there are some important differences of vocabulary which distinguish spoken from written language. There are some words and phrases you can happily say but you would never write, and there are some things you can read and write but never utter.

Standards and degrees of formality differ in speech and written English. Take the word 'though'. You might say 'I might ring him up,' and receive the answer 'Yes, you could but it wouldn't be very wise though because he hates the telephone.' Here *though* introduces an objection meant to outweigh the argument contained in the *yes*. But this does not go so well in the written form where *however* would be more appropriate. 'Yes, you could but it wouldn't be very wise, however' looks better.

It is, therefore, necessary for teachers both to compose useful work based on 'likely' English, rather than the beautifully grammatical, and to initiate the lipreader into the need for lipreading rapid, conversational English. I have found classes always responsive and extremely interested in such work. Adults should be very clear that every lesson is a step towards this goal and a teacher fully justify whatever she is doing, whether it be drill and the donkey work of any skill, or work on sentence composition.

There are many ways in which we can compose a sentence using the same words:

Occasionally I feel tired.

I occasionally feel tired.

I feel tired occasionally.

and

You ought to go to the Ritz some time.

You ought, sometime, to go to the Ritz.

Sometime you ought to go to the Ritz.

A lipreader does not know which composition is likely to be used and should, therefore, see and recognize all three patterns.

This is not an easy task for any teacher. Language is made up of words and English is generally agreed to be the richest of the world's languages. The Oxford English Dictionary lists nearly 415,000 words, about half of which are in common use. There are also 3,001,000 technical terms not found in ordinary dictionaries. English owes its large vocabulary to the fact that it can and has borrowed words adapted from other languages — jazz, aqualung, atomic, pop, satellite, bikini, ketchup, gingham, quartz — are examples; but few of us use more than a fraction of the words in the dictionary. Groucho Marx was once asked by a London newspaper to write a 2,000 word article for a fee of 200 dollars. He turned down the offer on the grounds that he already had 200 dollars but he was not sure he knew 2,000 words!

In fact, we all know a great deal more than that and most of use use about 8,000 words in ordinary conversation. A good journalist probably requires about 20,000 but Chaucer used only 8,000 because there were fewer words when he lived in the fourteenth century. To read *The Times* from cover to cover calls for a larger vocabulary of 50,000 because it involves special items such as ballet, scientific information, gardening and finance, but an everyday telephone conversation requires one-tenth of this number.

Another problem for the lipreader is that we are able to listen to people speaking at 322 words a minute (although it is more comfortable at 100), but for the eye to pick up fleeting shapes at the former speed would be impossible and even 100 words per minute would be daunting and exhausting for any lipreader. Apparently, we repeat ourselves, on average every 10 to 15 words and in conversation the word we use most is 'I', although in writing it becomes 'the'. We prefer to speak in monosyllables, such as yes, no, thanks, rather than in sentences, which is another drawback for a lipreader needing more words for extra clues. And, of course, words change in meaning over the years.

Adam (and we notice that he had speech) named the living creatures, not God, but hardly any thoughts ever made their way amongst mankind or assumed their proper importance unless, or until, selected words or phrases have nailed them down — today advertising does this extremely well. Originally the word 'lewd' meant lay, or unlearned, without any connotation of sin or distaste, and presumably 'awful' was 'full of awe' so that we might say, 'That beautiful sunset makes me feel awful'. And if a person has been deaf for the last thirty to forty years, there will have been many new words added to the language that he has never heard. Just consider the change in the word 'gay' in our lifetime.

Another useful point that emerged from the taping of conversations was that of the type of language most used colloquially — or what comes up most in everyday life? The greatest proportion of sentences were question forms, followed by explanations; then came diatribes or grumblings about something; and then the language of set situations, such as that used in talks, discussions and lectures. Such exercises give us useful indications as to the sort of lesson material that would be needed by a lipreading group.

Adult Learning

But before going on to present material, it is necessary to consider how adults learn. Socrates is usually the first teacher in people's minds when they speak of pedagogy. He first says that a teacher has no responsibility for the use to which a pupil puts his teaching. But he finally admits that in the end he would feel bound to give instruction in morals to a pupil who needed it, before putting into his hands the weapon of oratory. We must, therefore, give the deaf adult instruction on the uses and limitations of his skill before he learns it.

Adult learning is a pole apart from child learning. Children have the advantage of early mental growth and activity, when material learned is stored in the deep cortex of the brain and rarely forgotten, although it may become harder to recall with age. An adult comes with his learned knowledge, worldly experience, and reasoning powers, but his mode of learning will be almost impossible to change, as we find when trying to make an analytical learner into a synthetic one. A teacher is concerned with motivation, the pleasure principle and presentation, remembering that eye-plus-ear-plus-brain is lipreading and that we must present all variations on this in classes.

Is lipreading an art? Socrates notes that a genuine art is one which, like medicine or justice, employs a basis of knowledge to ensure the welfare of their objects and I like to think that lipreading also does this. So let us think on the principles of adult learning and try to apply these to the art of lipreading.

No skill is thoroughly learned and capable of immediate recall without *drill*, whether it be piano scales, or ballet steps, or throwing clay to make a pot. First, the lipreader must watch and concentrate on the speaker's face and be given watching practice. This may be done by drill on shapes in words — initial, middle and final consonants, and vowel changes — on different word shapes, changing the ending or start of a sentence, and on double consonants — to show the difference in p/pl/pr or f/fl/fr, for instance.

No skill is learned thoroughly without *repetition* — either of a common phrase, a progressive sentence or a similar build-up of a short piece of conversation or story.

A skill is more easily learned by *involvement* — this is not easily accomplished at the beginner's stage but it ensures the lipreader keeps his wits about him and starts to lipread other faces than the tutor's.

Material must be included for *mental stimulation* — to hold the interest, giving opportunities for making an intelligent guess, using subject matter that is forcing the lipreader to try the new skill.

A skill should be *pleasurable*. It may be difficult for someone to learn to skate but once the skill is mastered then it becomes a pleasure and a thrill. Can we give classes — even beginners — a chance to gain pleasure from their ability?

There should be *imaginative work* — a lipreader must learn to anticipate, to picture what verbal forms might be used in a given situation.

Like any skill, only a little is learned thoroughly at any one time and attention must be focused on the points to be made in each lesson and these revised from time to time if necessary.

Also, and this is equally important for hearing aid wearers, *listening practice* should be part of every session so that the lipreader learns to make full use of his aid and also use any residual hearing to its fullest extent.

A Brief Summary

To summarize points so far:

Language is designed for the *ear* and not the *eye*.

Who needs lipreading? Probably everyone — we all need to watch faces when in a noisy environment; all deafened adults with a 20 decibel loss or more; and, of course, those so deaf that they are entirely dependent on visual clues to understand speech.

What is lipreading? It is a skill requiring constant practice, good teaching and/or a natural ability with all the humps, pitfalls and disappointments of learning any skill.

We are fortunate to be English-speaking. A gutteral language, or one using back consonants, would be extremely difficult to lipread, as would one which relies on variations in pitch for meaning. The deafened adult usually loses the high tones of speech first, which involves missing the softer consonants, f, s, sh, but many retain hearing for the grosser, louder vowel sounds. In a sentence such as, 'Paul threw the ball out of the window,' the vowels or, oo, a, or, ow, o, a, i, o, would be heard, making not the slightest sense to the listener, but by learning and watching for the shapes made by P-thr-, th-, b-ll-t-f, th-, w-d, the two sets of clues can be amalgamated to make sense.

Lipreading Skill

I never cease to be amazed by the skill of many lipreaders. Most do not stop to consider what it is they are doing, they are probably too busy concentrating on the matter in hand; but working with individuals it has been possible to try to get them to think out what is happening when they appear to understand something which a teacher would consider impossible to lipread.

I recall telling a client an item I had read in a newspaper that week, feeling certain that she would miss the final sentence. The article concerned a visit by the Queen Mother to open a new hospital wing. A small boy had been chosen to present a bouquet and, having handed this to the Queen Mother, he couldn't contain himself. He said to her, 'Mam, I know your daughter — she's the Queen.' 'Yes,' said the Queen Mother, smiling at him, 'Isn't it exciting!'

Watch yourself saying this sentence, as quietly as possible, looking into a mirror and you will see nothing more than a few jogs of the teeth, but this lipreader told me exactly what it was. When I asked her to think how she had lipread that, her reply was, 'I could tell by your expression — you *looked* excited,' strengthening my belief that lipreading is dependent on many other clues besides lip movements.

It is possible to attain such a high standard of skill that such small differences as word stress, prefixes and slight changes in sentence structure can be distinguished. Differences in such phrases as:

I can hear.
I can, here.

The whirl of tomorrow.
The world of tomorrow.

I wish for happiness most of the time.
I wish for ham and eggs most of the time.

Shall we eat grandmother?
Shall we eat, grandmother?

There will always be phrases that are indistinguishable even to the best lipreader. Is it, 'He's disgusted with me,' or 'He discussed it with me'? And the woman who read, 'It distresses me when my corsets are new' for, 'It distresses me when my daughters argue,' was mentally tuned in to do so, since she had bought herself a new pair which were tormenting her and that was in the forefront of her mind!

Facial Expressions

Can you learn to lipread punctuation? That is, can you lipread expression caused by change in voice? The full stop and the question mark and the exclamation mark are there to show us, when reading, to make a voice change. The phrase 'Jones has scored' would be said as a flat statement, but 'Jones has scored?' would need a different intonation, which would result in facial muscles being brought into play, and 'Jones has scored!' might even involve eye muscles — all valuable clues to a lipreader.

It is difficult to distinguish two monkeys just by observing their faces, since a monkey has few facial muscles and can do little more than express rage or fright. Humans have muscles in their faces that enable them to wink, to blink, to screw up their eyes, frown, raise eyebrows, wrinkle noses, sniff, snort, grimace, smile, pout, simper, look dismal, happy, peeved, and so on. Each set of movements helps to provide a clue as to a person's mood and likely use of language.

In 1977 two British scientists put forward some very unexpected results concerning the roles of eyes and ears in perceiving speech. Harry Gurk and J. Macdonald, of the University of Surrey, had noticed that dubbed films often seemed funny, given the poor fit of lips and sounds. They made a video tape that showed the face of a woman saying either 'Ba' or 'Pa'. But they dubbed a new sound track over the visual display in which the voice said 'Ga' or 'Ka'. The researchers believed that the eyes would not fool the ears. They expected that people who viewed these videos, or listened to them with their eyes shut, would not have their perception of speech altered. So that if the tape said 'Ba' then the subjects would hear 'Ba', irrespective of the lip movements of the woman on the screen.

I remember going to one of these demonstrations, where about fourteen professionals were asked to watch the screen and listen. When we just heard the sounds of 'Ba', or 'Ga', or 'Pa', or 'Ka', we made hardly any errors but seeing 'tricked' lips led to mistakes. When the lips showed 'Ga' and the sound said 'Ba', then the majority of adults heard 'Da'. In other words, the two conflicting perceptions are fused by the brain into quite a different one, and this surely is a point we must remember when dealing with the deaf, who receive one distortion through an aid and see a differing pattern on the lips.

At first Gurk and MacDonald thought this phenomenon applied only to a consonant plus vowel, but then they generated series of lip movements for a sentence, accompanied by a different sentence on the tape, and most subjects heard a third version which they were adamant was correct. In other words, it wasn't just an effect at the start of a word but applied also to end sounds and whole sentences. Their hypothesis was that the ear picks up such information as to whether a consonant is voiced or voiceless, whether it is a nasal or a fricative, while the eye is picking up the place where the articulation occurs. Then, during the processing of the clues, these two bits of information are put together and you get the resolution — which is an illusion. The researchers hoped that their work would not only help us to understand more about the interpretation of speech, but actually help teach the deaf to make better use of the speech perception they have.

Cued Speech
Another interest for the hard of hearing is the method of Cued Speech, designed to assist lipreaders in deciphering those movements which cause confusion, that is the pairing of sounds which make similar shapes, e.g. (p b), (f v), (t d).

These were thought out by Dr R. Orin Cornett and an English version was adapted because of the vowel differences in English/American speech. The classes in the Centre for the Deaf were asked whether they would welcome this system but the feeling, without exception, was that any form of signing was abhorrent and no one wished to learn the cueing system. I accept this point but, on the other hand, have often suggested to couples, or to professionals who have a secretary working for them, that it takes very little time to use the old English finger alphabet, and the occasional use of one of these movements would save time and frustration. For example, many words contain the unlipreadable prefixes, con/ir/il/dis, and one finger movement to denote each of these is helpful in conveying a rapid meaning.

Visualizing Speech

Let us look now at the letters we know and try to visualize what we might hope to see or miss in analysing speech. Mirror practice is sometimes suggested for those unable to attend classes. Although I believe this to have an extremely limited use in learning the skill, which requires constant practice from the lips of others, it is useful to see yourself make these shapes into a mirror and so help to learn the elements of what you might expect to see on other lips.

One of the most difficult early points is for a lipreader to forget the 'name' of each letter and think of it as a sound. For instance, the letter b is actually a word — bee or be; the letter c is see or sea; d is dee and f is ef and so on. So that when spelling a word such as Phyllis you would name the letters, pea, aitch, why, double ell, eye, ess. The lipreader is required to forget the name and think of ph as f, y as short vowel i, the two lls as one, the i as a short vowel made inside the mouth, and the s as a slight movement of the lips.

So, initially, practice is given on watching the shape that letters make.

Visible consonants are those which the lipreader can see clearly:

p, b, m: need to be thought of together since they look virtually the same in words, although the person wearing an aid might well distinguish the voice used in making b and nasality of m. The lips meet, close and part with some explosion of air. They are easily recognizable but cause confusion, as words such as pier, peer, beer, bier, and mere, will look alike. However, this problem is often overrated. With skill, the lipreader is less likely to confuse such words when in context and is more likely to make mistakes with other words which look very unlike in the written form, yet are difficult to distinguish on the lips. 'Day' and 'night' are examples of this.

f and *v*:   look the same, being made with the same lip movement; the upper teeth meet with the lower lip and part. This will make words such as fail, vale, and veil, look alike but there are so many more words that begin with f that it is more likely to be this letter. It is more likely that readers will make mistakes over words such as visitor and friend than the true homophenes.

w, wh, qu: all made by a close rounding of the lips. Wh resembles w, because the h is merely breath which is taken before the shaping for w — we should write it as hw! Few words start with qu, but it is possible to read white instead of quite.

r: a book on speech production will show many different forms of this consonant but the accepted shape, full face view, is that the corners of the mouth are puckered and move in, lips are slightly pouting. The pouting is more obvious with a side view.

On poor speakers the lipreader may mistake r for w, or ch.

sh, ch, j: and the noise found in the middle of a word such as leisure or pleasure. These have the same visual shape, with the pouting lips, and soft g looks like this too. Share and chair would look alike, or choke and joke, and it should be remembered that the same shapes as final consonants will cause a similar confusion e.g. ba*sh* bat*ch* bad*ge*.

s, z, and soft *c*: are placed here with the visible consonants since there is mouth movement, although the sibilant sound presents a very small shape. The teeth are together, or almost shut, and lips are usually spread (although not always when a vowel with liprounding comes before or after). To see what is happening for s it is good practice to watch yourself say first arm then arms, and then eat, reheat then reseat.

h: is breath only, so has no visual shape of its own. It takes on the shape of the following vowel. This means that am looks like ham and edge looks like hedge. You have to rely on guesswork for this letter but context will show that this is not difficult. For example, 'I'm always ill after walking up that hill,' and 'There is a hedge at the edge of the field.' And I doubt that we would say, 'When I am hungry I fancy a ham sandwich,' since we would probably contract the 'I am' to 'I'm'.

H is more of a problem when it appears in the middle of a word so that reheat could be reseat and rehash mistaken for rash.

l: should be easier to see since the tongue flashes up to the front palate and down. But when l does not appear at the end or the start of a word, then the tongue is brought back, resulting in the 'dark' l which may be confused with the movement made by n.

th: really has two sounds, both voiced and voiceless, e.g. *th*e *th*umb. But it is one of the easiest shapes to see. The tongue tip can be seen between the upper and lower teeth (teeth gently touch the tongue tip).

t, d: some teachers will add n to this pairing but this can cause confusion to the hearing aid user, who will possibly be able to hear the nasal sound. Also, in speech teaching, the movements for td and n are entirely different. They are all difficult to see. For td, in a good light and with a clear speaker, the tongue tip may be seen to go up and behind the top front teeth, where it is quickly flicked and comes away. Teeth are usually slightly parted but these sounds may be said with the mouth shut, so that the tongue movement cannot be seen.

There are other consonants which are made inside the mouth and therefore do not appear as lip movements:
c, k, ck: as in cuff, keep, and flick. Possible clues are a slight movement under and behind the chin and a slight 'gap' in the word in some cases.

n, -ng, -ing: are nasal sounds. Sometimes the tongue may be seen held back to close the throat and prevent air leaving the mouth. Words containing these sounds may be guessed from context by the good lipreader, e.g. I ra dow the road, is unlikely to cause a problem. Even when two of these sounds come together, as in br*inging* or cl*inging*, contextual guidance will overcome the invisibility. For instance, 'the birds were s------ at five o'clock this morning,' will be guessed.

y: is difficult to see and describe since it is properly a combination of vowels, ee + a, as in yellow, usual, and Euston. It is normally recognized because there are few words with this shape. In some words there is a decided down movement of the lower jaw.

x: is a combination of sounds, eks, or may be said as z, as in Xerox. It is best taught as part of a lesson on k, or s/z, or as the prefix ex- for the better lipreaders.

These consonantal shapes should be practised to excess, since most of these give body to a sentence and make our language intelligible. Many 'speed reading' systems are based on ignoring the vowels in a word and reading consonants only, so that it is possible to read the following line without effort and with speed: Th gvrnmnt hs dcdd t stp ll pymnts fr th tm bng. There are at least two books on the market written entirely in consonants which are quite readable.

Before considering the vowels of speech let us look at a few ways in which we might learn one of the consonantal shapes, and take one of the easiest to see — f.

To give some watching practice
Look at the start of these words   *f*ill *f*or *f*ate while they are repeated several times

Now look at the end of these words   ti*ff* roo*f* mu*ff*

Now pick it out of the middle of these words   pre*f*er re*f*it tele*ph*one — ph will also be like f.

The Long vowels are low frequency sounds which may well be heard by the hearing aid user and which are therefore invaluable aids to making sense of speech. Although we have seen that it is the consonants which give language intelligibility, the vowels give us the flow and rhythm of speech which makes every sentence a pattern. It is important for lipreaders who still hear sound to practise sentences differing in rhythm and stress.

There are five long vowels and it is worth looking at the shapes each one makes as well as trying to listen to their sounds.

ah: as pronounced in farm, calm, path, and heart, has a fairly wide jaw opening, with the lips neutral, i.e. neither spread nor rounded.

oo: as pronounced in boon, jewel, route, suit, and lute has a narrow jaw opening, with the lips closely rounded.

er: as pronounced in fern, bird, worm, earth, myrhh, and turn. The jaw opening is medium, with the lips neutral or slightly pouting.

aw: as pronounced in law, bore, door, four, and war, has the jaw opening fairly wide and open lip-rounding.

ee: as pronounced in see, be, feat, key, and mete, has a very narrow mouth opening, with the lips spread, and is the most difficult to distinguish.

As for the *short vowels*, there are seven, including the neutral as in *a*bout, and it is possible to show lipreaders that they do make differing shapes just by drilling from tip, top, and tap, but they are normally lost for the lipreader who is coping with running speech.

There are *dipthongs*, which show more movement since the mouth moves from one vowel to another, as when we say the word 'boy' or 'here' or 'play', and then there are triple sounds in such words as 'fire' and 'power' and 'player'. But if the lipreader wishes to know of these, there are many excellent speech therapy books which give complete lists of such sounds. I have not found that dealing with phonetics is of very much use in lipreading — it is of more value to practise everyday phrases and sentences as these would commonly be said, rather than to try and break down speech into its constituents. Few people, for example, use triphthongs when they speak and actually pronounce all three vowels of 'mower' or '(em)ployer'.

Sounds are assimilated when we speak, unless we are very pedantic speakers and deliberately finish off each word and separate this from the next. Most people would say 'Don't worry about him, he'll be alright,' rather than 'Do not' and 'he will'. 'Do you want to come out for a walk?' is more likely to come out as, 'Jew want to come fra walk?' and this is what the lipreader will see, *not* perfectly articulated spoken language.

Therefore, to summarize, before we consider how we might train the hearing we still possess, here are suggestions to give a lipreader the best possible conditions for understanding speech:

1. Have the light behind you, falling on the speaker's

face, to help you see clearly.

2.   Be prepared to ask the speaker to remove a cigarette from his mouth, or slow down a little.

3.   Try to sit or stand on the same level, so that you are face to face with the speaker.

4.   Try to pick out some words so that you can ask 'Did you say ...?' rather than 'What did you say?' as people soon grow irritated at repeating all they have said.

5.   Keep your hearing aid in good order by having it checked regularly.

Do not expect to hear everyone and understand everything. Even those with good hearing often have to make a guess or just get the gist of what has been said.

Sound is a peculiar property. You will hear some voices better than others — this will depend on your hearing loss and the speaker's tone of voice.

Sound will be better in certain rooms — churches, large empty rooms or tiled areas will make sound hollow or reverberating.

Do not expect sympathy and understanding from everyone. Deafness can be irritating, requiring patience and understanding from all parties concerned. People with normal hearing often have problems in noisy situations but, of course, yours is with you all the time, and this is hard for hearing people to imagine.

To the helper: Patience, sympathy and understanding are essential. If you leave out the first two you would not be able to hope to increase the understanding. However, this sounds glib advice when faced with deafness, either a deaf member of the family, a co-worker, or a friend. There is no disgrace on either side if a written word has to be used — I always have a pad or two handy when entertaining deaf friends, knowing that the deaf person will not lipread all I say and I shall find it a strain, after a time, trying to think of different ways of repeating myself.

Communication is the be-all. What is important is tact and sensitivity — to know when resorting to writing would relieve strain, and not to monopolize the conversation so that the lipreader is forced to work hard all the time.

Remember that the deaf cannot drink and eat and watch at the same time.

Remember not to shout — it is of no help to the totally deaf and, to the hearing aid wearer, only adds distortion to the sounds he is receiving.

If you are a person who uses gestures, then keep these to a minimum, away from your face, and try to make them meaningful. The lipreader cannot watch your mouth movements and your hands at the same time.

Try not to show irritation or impatience in your face. Instead think of another way you might express what you have said and try again, remembering the sentence you just used might be unlipreadable.

Remember that the hearing aid is magnifying all sounds within earshot, so carrying on a conversation at the side of a traffic flow is difficult on both sides. The totally deaf person will manage to lipread, since he is not put out by the noise, but the speaker will probably start to shout to hear himself and exaggerate his lip movements. If the deaf person wears an aid then horrible sounds from passing traffic, greatly magnified, will be preventing him from lipreading — so try to go off into a side road if it is important that you converse.

Remember above all that you may now have good hearing yourself but, even if an old age deafness is all you are likely to suffer later on, you will need all the consideration and sympathetic understanding that a deaf person needs now, and that seems little enough to give to someone denied the pleasant ease of conversation and exchange of ideas.

5

PITFALLS FOR THE HARD OF HEARING

in every language even deafanddumb
thy sons acclaim your glorious name by gorry
by jingo by gee by gosh by gum

e.e. cummings

First of all, I would like to repeat the point that all practice must be useful general language and give some examples of the pitfalls *and* aids that the deaf can make work for them. Deaf people might be called 'absurd' since this is derived from a Latin word meaning deaf, dulled. In fact the French call their deaf 'les surds'. Yet it is our language that is absurd in the modern sense, being at times incongruous and unreasonable.

I feel that lipreaders can only acquire their skill through observation of the ordinary and the obvious, and learning something that Whitman called 'the profound lesson of reception'. Naturally it helps to acquire the visible shapes of single sounds as a foundation for speech recognition, yet there is little enough to see at times and still lipreaders are able to grasp a meaning. New words and new slang flow into the language all the time; much of the older slang lingers on even though its origins are forgotten; and there are always new books appearing discussing the state of the language — most of them extremely interesting and just the sort of literature to take on desert islands. What I am endeavouring to promote is a mode of teaching based on language, rather than an analytical review of sound shapes. Sounds change in shape when in the rhythm of a sentence so that although drill is a necessary principle for learning, teaching sounds in isolation is less useful than teaching them in likely combinations of language. As a simple example, in the sentence:

It makes me mad — when I think of all the money she wastes. Or,
It makes me see red — when I think of all the money she wastes.

We can certainly agree that m is a good shape to see — then we must remember that too many like shapes are confusing to the eye. Just try saying 'We will wash with warm water' to a group of lipreaders and, despite the fact that you have told them that w is a good visible shape, they will find the sentence a problem. For this reason, sentences taken from a book on speech therapy are not ideal for lipreading practice since they are based on a different practice premise — to be able to *say* the same sound many times, as in 'Betty Botter bought some butter'. We must, therefore, either use the entire phrase 'It makes me mad' or 'It makes me see red' for the lipreader to gain a picture from the rhythm, or we must suggest that they let the eye swan over the difficulty and concentrate on any clues appearing later in the sentence, or look for additional visual clues such as the mood of the speaker. We must also see that practice is given on varying the position of the phrase in the sentence — it might come at the end, 'When I see her wasting money — it makes me mad.' So often it is the start of a sentence that is said rapidly and often that has few lipreadable shapes, just look at yourself saying in a very quiet voice, 'Isn't it odd...' 'I bet he...' 'Did he tell you...' 'It's about time we...' 'Did you get...'.

Therefore, although it does not mean that we have to be completely permissive about language, we cannot deplore jargon and bad grammar and expressions such as 'ongoing' and 'going spare' while these are being used by people. There is good and bad use of English at many levels, and different English for varying situations, and we can do no more than accept that we cannot reform language and offer our clients English 'as she is spoke', rather than as one would wish it to be spoken and written.

An American teacher had her greatest success with a group of war veterans who had to learn to lipread as quickly as possible in order to return to other posts in the services. She worked in small groups, getting them to talk clearly to each other, standing by to pick up difficulties and drilling these immediately, and it is said that she was able to return the men to their jobs within a few weeks. They were plunged in at the deep end and, we must remember an important point, they had every incentive to learn. But lipreading can be mastered reasonably quickly if all conditions are right — lessons based on learning principles, plenty of drill on common phrases, motivation, and checking all the time that progress *is* being made.

If the deaf, or the hard of hearing, are confronted with the problems they will appreciate what they have to do. I once had a pedantic speaker in a group who declared that people always said 'I will' and 'We would not' (and it is likely that in his particular circle people did), until I showed him a birthday card I received one day. The front showed a creature looking at three rows of very healthy looking lettuces. Turning to the inner page was just the phrase, 'Lettuce wish you a Happy Birthday'. The client thought this extremely funny and somehow it made the point to him that we do use phrases that sound very much alike, and therefore look alike, because we don't articulate every sound and syllable.

Language Fun

Words are so interesting that it is possible to make an entire lesson on a few examples. For example, the English word 'head' and the Latin 'caput' derive from a common Indo-European root. Head still retains its primitive meaning in English, but the French altered 'caput' to 'chief' and brought this to England where it became chief with the meaning of head, e.g. head of an army. For the English this widened the meaning of head and now we can say head of an army or chief of an army as we please; and we prefer to use Headmaster instead of chiefmaster.

Take a simple schoolboy joke, 'What's the greatest feat in eating ever known?' 'Well, there was once a man who started by bolting a door, then he threw up a window and after that he sat down and swallowed, a whole storey.' There is enough material there to give practice; showing that was/once start with similar shapes; that greatest/feat/ eating show different sounds; that threw/through and story/storey are homophenous; and going on to words used in eating, hungry, starving, glutton, finicky, greedy,

epicure, gourmand, anorexic, obese, trying to cover at least
a part of the situational English used about food and eating
habits.

It is good to encourage a quick response. Some words go
naturally together and are known to most English people.
Speed can be attained by asking a lipreader to give the final
word of phrases such as:

Red, white and ...
A hop, a skip and a ...
Fee, fi, fo, ...
Faith, hope and ...
Tinker, tailor, soldier ...
Healthy, wealthy and ...
Silk, satin, cotton ...
Animal, vegetable and ...
This, that and ...
Head, heart and ...
Blood, toil, sweat and ...

Another amazing ability is how quickly people are able to
give the name of a sport after hearing only two or three
words. I think this is very good practice in as much as a
lipreader is always trying to come to a conclusion from very
little in the way of clues.

The lipreader should be shown the idea first — that
certain words are common to an activity or a situation; in
this case, a sport, so that if I say, ring, glove, sponge, canvas,
then boxing is the sport connected with these four words.
For example:

Racquet, ball, court, net, umpire,
board, pieces, knight, pawn,
pitch, referee, whistle, goal, penalty,
board, score, throw, bull, darts,
course, horses, tote, grandstand, stalls.

Other such lists can be tried.

I recall walking along a platform in the Underground one
morning. Standing on the platform was a woman porter in
uniform and walking towards her was a male fellow
worker. He was munching a Mars bar and as he drew nearer
she called out to him, 'Gis a bit'. I went on my way
thinking, 'Well, I would be standing in front of a group of
lipreaders saying "The g in give is not visible but look for

the v as this is a splendid clue,'' ' — only to find that in everyday speech a large proportion of speakers would not even be making the v. The spoken word really is very different from the written. There is a rhythm and tempo for speaking and quite another for writing and we can no more accommodate both simultaneously than Fred Astaire could dance a foxtrot and tango at the same time.

A word will change its meaning depending merely on its position in a sentence:

The nurse *only* broke her wrist. (She didn't lose it altogether.)

Only the nurse broke her wrist (Nobody else suffered.)

The only nurse broke her wrist (So no other nurses could.)

The nurse broke only her wrist (Nothing else suffered.)

Commonly in language we use two statements, one being the cause of the other, and these are of help to a lipreader in as much as there is a chance of lipreading enough of the first or second part, and then being able to make sense of the other. The mind often seems to work backwards and lipreaders usually say, when asked how they understood, 'Well I got the last part and then the first clicked for me'. The following sentences show examples of this practice:

'She has a very bad cold. She can hardly speak.'

'We saw a great many places on our holiday. I can't remember half of them.'

'I've just bought some more bread. I didn't want to be short over the holiday weekend.'

'No buses run at this time of night. We shall have to ring for a taxi.'

Or sometimes the lipreader must be prepared for a statement followed by a question:

'I'm going to the meeting tomorrow — are you?'

'I haven't heard from them for several years — have you?'

'I can't find my doorkey anywhere — have you seen it?'

'I can come next Friday — where shall we meet?'

Question forms are not always at the start of sentences and quite often it is not the questioning word, such as what? which? why?, that is the problem but the entire phrase, so that it is more useful to practise such colloquial instances as:

'What are you going to do about...?'
'Will he be able to...?'
'What time's the...?
'Why are you...?'
'Where d'you think...?

Even more important, there are questions which do not have a lipreadable question form to start with, that is those that start with 'Did' or 'Can' or 'Is it'. These also should be contrasted with the negatives, 'Didn't' and 'Can't' and 'Isn't it'.

Language is situational or episodic. It is an imaginative exercise to ask a lipreader to put himself into a situation and imagine what might be said to him. For example, imagine you are sweeping leaves away from the front of your house. A passer-by might stop and say in passing any of the following remarks:

'Rather you than me!'
'You've got a never-ending job there!' or 'You've got a thankless job there!'
'I'd let the wind blow them somewhere else if I were you!'
'Aren't they a nuisance!'
'Good job you don't have to count them all, isn't it!'
'You'll have a lovely lot of compost from that lot!'
'You need a Hoover for all those!'
Even, from a joker, 'If I were you I'd *leave* well alone!'

There are many points here to note. First, no reply is necessary. If the remark has not been lipread then a smile or a nod covers the situation. Then, does emphasis help? Is it possible to get a voice clue from the exclamations? Notice also that language is left out in everyday speech, 'What a' is understood before the phrase starting, 'Good job...' and, finally, there is no mention of the subject under discussion by name (leaves).

It is worthwhile thinking about and practising the type of language someone is likely to use in certain situations — what a visitor might say when he arrives, what an acquaintance in the street is likely to say, what a stranger in the street is likely to say, what your partner is likely to say when she returns from shopping or seeing a friend, and the scores of other daily events in our lives.

To be imaginative is part of the way to being able to anticipate. Of course you might be wrong, but if you are don't ask, 'What did you say?' or you will be given the same unlipreadable pattern; ask, 'Did you say "The moon is made from green cheese?" ' and then you will get, 'No I said...' which at least gives you a second chance and perhaps a slightly changed version this time.

The deafened adult has the enormous advantage over the born deaf of having acquired natural language and being well aware of suitable retorts and sentences likely to be used in a given situation. His problem is having to recognize this language is a new form through visual shapes, a hearing aid, or other clues, and he is unable to prevent hearing people from using words that they like the sound of, or using words they like, without much care for their meaning. His one hope is to watch and read and keep abreast of fresh phrases and 'in' words and, possibly, at the same time gain fresh insight and interest for the richness of our own tongue.

6

LISTENING PRACTICE

I must first state that this is not what is meant professionally by auditory training. The latter will be training carried out with machines that both amplify and select sound, with graded tapes of balanced word lists, and by a professional worker who can prepare work suitable for an individual hearing loss. However, since it is most important that the lipreader use his remaining hearing in conjunction with his visual skill, the following material can be used by a helper in a similar way to the lipreading practice notes. One important difference is that these listening sessions should be kept short — it is far more tiring to hear distorted sound than it is to lipread — and the helper must either make a note or remember what sounds the lipreader finds most difficult and try to give much repetition on these. The helper will not know exactly what it is the lipreader is hearing and it is, therefore, essential that the lipreader *always* repeats what he thinks he has heard.

As in lipreading, the reader will use his knowledge of language to fill in blanks to make sense of something. But the main aim of this practice is to keep the hearer listening to sounds of speech, to help him in discriminating these, and to maintain a memory of everyday noises so that he will remain stimulated through sound and make full use of his aid and any residual hearing he possesses. The helper might devise his own methods of doing this — just a simple exercise of sitting opposite the listener, telling him to shut his eyes or look away, and doing such actions as clapping his hands, stamping his feet, banging on the table, coughing, blowing his nose, sighing, and asking the listener to distinguish what he is doing. This makes for concentration on the source of a sound and is basic to any listening practice. It is not a waste of time but a means of making certain that a deafened adult uses all means open to him to ease a communication problem.

Before You Start

Sit opposite each other and have some rough paper to make notes or confirm material. The listener should have his aid on normal setting. The helper should speak in a level, clear, steady voice; enunciation must be particularly exact but without exaggeration — for example, if you try to emphasize the endings of words, such as rub, or rap, then you will find that you are adding the neutral vowel and rub will sound like rubber and rap like wrapper. Even if you have to give the word several times try not to over-emphasize or slow the syllables, as this will change the rhythm of the word or phrase.

Part of the aim is for the deafened adult to learn the weak spots in his hearing and at which distance he hears best. If he is doing very well at a close range then try the material at a further distance, a foot further away at a time. As the listener grows in confidence then try adding a little background noise from a radio. The listener might find that he benefits from Willis' paracusis, which is a term used by physicians to describe the phenomenon by which certain hard of hearing people seem to hear much better in noisy places like restaurants and machine shops. If the listener has the type of deafness involving only the middle ear then he may get on quite well with the noise, but if he suffers from deafness involving the nerve centres of the ear then he will experience a lot of difficulty in noisy places. Even though people speaking to him raise their voices this makes it no easier for him to understand and often causes even more problems of confusion. So if your listener actively dislikes any background do not introduce this.

It may be found that the listener prefers to shift his head and favour one ear more than the other. This is because if he has normal hearing on one side and impairment on the other he will complain of direction-finding disability. There is a difference in sound pressure between one ear and the other, created by the sound shadow of diffraction of sound around the head and a person with a loss in one ear will develop a knack of turning the head quickly in order to locate sounds more easily. In fact it is a good exercise to make loud sounds in a corner of a room behind the listener's head, to give him time to observe this direction finding phenomenon.

The listener should get into the habit of noting down every word or letter which he finds difficult to hear, or which he misses and supplies later from the sense of the sentence. In this way it becomes possible to isolate and work on specific sounds and words. You may find that your listener never hears any of the high soft speech sounds — the f, s, and th — which means that even his aid is not able to amplify these sounds sufficiently for him to hear them, or the nerve ending that responds to that frequency has been destroyed. In this case he will have to rely on context to complete a sentence and any drills using these sounds must be left out, since with these he has no contextual guidance. He needs a fairly long phrase or sentence to provide other clues.

Understanding Speech

After the Second World War the American government faced the problem of returning veterans who had suffered hearing losses. These men were sent to free centres, and provided with aids and tutors to teach them lipreading and to put them through a period of auditory re-training. The experience gained in this rehabilitation showed that it was possible to train deafened individuals to make far more effective use of any hearing that remained. They were taught to understand speech better, even though they heard only a fraction of what a normal ear would hear, by re-educating the hearing centres. Most of us are born with the ability to perceive *sounds* but the ability to understand *speech* is an ability which has to be acquired.

Children need years of listening to speech and associating certain words with certain objects, people and situations until the words become familiar and meaningful. When adults listen to a foreign tongue, which they do not know, this pattern of sound has no association in their mind; but if they go to live in that country then slowly some words become meaningful and after several years they will possibly become quite fluent in understanding the language. Let us then suppose that these people move away from that country and no longer hear this second tongue they have learned. The memory of this language will start to fade and the hearing centres in the brain become indistinct for this second language. When they hear this language again at some later date they will find it difficult to understand, because they have lost this sound vocabulary. Then, by re-using this almost forgotten tongue, they will gradually again become familiar with it and relearn it much more quickly the second time around, but it will still require a lot of study. The person who loses hearing can be compared to someone who no longer hears a once-familiar language. He receives only a fraction of the practice in hearing spoken words that normal hearing people get.

As the degree of hearing loss increases, and fewer speech sounds are heard, a habit of inattention may occur — after all, what is the use of constantly straining to understand if speech is so unclear that it might as well be a foreign language? In most cases, the loss of discrimination is gradual but the ability to understand remains intact and practice can be given to re-establish half-forgotten sounds. As with lipreading, it is a matter of practice, repetition, and working at it, and the suggested exercises are a beginning in the task of re-familiarizing the listener with sounds which have lost meaning and the patterns of everyday speech. We must remember that most of our comprehension of language is not actually of individual words but of the tenor of a phrase and this is related to what each of us anticipates from experience, what we desire to hear or even what we presume will be heard next.

When we introduce a listening practice it is usual to start with gross sounds, such as the loud vowel sounds as they appear in single words, but it is imperative that we also give practice in sentence forms and dialogue and stories, so that the person with the more severe loss can then relate clues to language. These practice pieces are short because I believe professional help is essential for intense auditory training, but this is not to say that much useful work can be done with a helper who is willing to work through the suggested material. Any practice which improves concentration and keeps the deafened adult concentrating on sound is invaluable.

Working Alone

If it is not possible to find a member of the family or a friend able to offer listening practice there is a way of helping yourself. There are lists of several hundreds of the most common English words — they appear in books on typing and office practice, in Pitman manuals, and sometimes in English books. You can train your sound memory on this list by picking out a random group of five or six words. Write these down and repeat each word aloud. Then turn the list over and repeat them aloud from memory. If you should ever have a helper then they can repeat the few words to you — start with three and work up to five or more as your memory for the sounds improves. Then after completing several such groups (remember to tick off those you have tried), try increasing the speed of delivery.

In similar vein, listen to a speaker on radio or television with the volume adjusted so that the speech is audible. Listen to a sentence at a time and then turn down the volume control and see if you can repeat the sentence *exactly* as you heard it. That is true listening.

The Vowels

Vowels are important because these are the strong elements of speech and they are generally lower in pitch, so that many adults who still have useful residual hearing will hear most or all of them.

Another reason for trying to listen to the vowels is because they are the more difficult to lipread, especially the short vowels. True they make large or broad shapes in isolation, but this openness is often not seen in running speech. Listen as the helper reads the following to you and repeat back:

barn	burn	boon
boon	born	barn
born	been	burn
bird	board	bead
booed	bead	bard

She picked up the bird.
She picked up the board.
She picked up the bead.

These two simple exercises should be done several times

until the listener is sure of long vowel differences. The reader should repeat slowly to begin with and then increase speed. The listener must hear each one several times to hold a sound pattern in his head — he will often ask to hear one or two over again — so give a lot of repetition and mix the order sometimes.

Numbers

Numbers can often be identified by the vowel even when the consonant is inaudible. The following list shows what the vowel sounds are like in numbers:

One — uh
Two — oo
Three — ee
Four — aw
Five — eye
Six — ih
Seven — eh...eh
Eight — ay
Nine — eye
Ten — eh

You will hear that five and nine have the same vowel sound, but the lipreader would use his knowledge of shape to distinguish them and it is likely that the hearing aid wearer would also hear the nasal ending of number nine. It is worth trying to pick out some numbers from sentences:

The number of my house is seven.
They have two bathrooms.
I shall be about five minutes.
I'm going away in three days time.
Did you say he is ten this month?
They have four boys and one girl.
The train was eight minutes late.
We picked nine pounds of cherries from our tree.
He won't be home until after six.

Similarities and Differences

Practice may be given in listening for the similarities and differences in phrases. To begin it is better to use only two sentences and then progress to using three. The sentences should each be read twice and then one chosen to repeat and the listener asked which it is.

He's being very hard.
He's being very harsh.

Doesn't she grow!
Doesn't she glow!

She's no lady.
She's not lazy.

I'm leaving with my brother.
I'm living with my brother.

The water is coming from a lake.
The water is coming from a leak.

The strain is terrible.
The terrain is terrible.

What a chain of events!
What a change of events!

He came in late.
He came in laden.

You ought to feel it.
You ought to fill it.

She's making beads for the shop.
She's making bids for the shop.

He lent me his coat.
He lent me his boat.

This is the right place.
This is the light case.
This is the right case.

He claims it's your ball.
He claims it's your call.
We came for your ball.

That's a very low tune.
That's a slow tune.
That's a very low tone.

I want the long knife.
I want a long life.

You seemed so strange.
You seemed so strained.
You seemed so distrait.

He looked through the last door.
He looked through the glass door.
He pushed through the glass door.

I have no wish to fill this book with exercises on all vowels, consonants, and other more complex speech sounds. There are many excellent books on speech therapy which contain these. Not everyone uses the same vowel sounds in words — many Northern speakers make little use of some short vowels and substitute long ones in words such as book, food and pull, and these must be regarded as dialect substitutions, not errors. In books on speech therapy exercises will be given on words containing each sound of speech, also phrases using the sound. However, these are for *speech* training and sentences such as, 'She says she can sew a sheet,' and 'Put the cut pumpkin in a pipkin,' although excellent tongue manipulators, are not the language heard in normal living conditions. Sample exercises shown here are meant to sustain *interest* in the listening situation and encourage the element of putting two and two together, essential for understanding.

Some of the exercises may require a little effort in writing out a few cards, but this need be done only as roughly as is legible — their use is to give the listener some focal point while concentrating since he cannot be expected to hold nine or ten sentences in his head. For example, practise can be given in listening to a voiced and its equivalent unvoiced sound. Back consonants, such as k and g, are not lipreadable but it is possible that an aural clue will be heard. The voiced g will be louder than k and if the helper will write the following sentences on slips of paper or card he can repeat them and ask the listener to point to the one selected, and do this several times on different occasions:

Can you come with me tomorrow? Can you go with me tomorrow?

It would be good if you could come too. Would you be good enough to come too?

He carried a large crate. He carried a great box.

The addition of a little sound at the start of a word might be missed. So practise:
    sleep/asleep
    specially/especially
    reverently/irreverently
    The matter was specially/especially interesting to him.
    Did you see him sleep/asleep on the lawn?
    He spoke most reverently/irreverently about it.
    It is greed/It is agreed.

This little sound may occur in the middle of a word. Listen to:
    pens/pennies sport/support blow/below mint/minute
    What sport/support is available?
    Can you lend me some pens/pennies?
    I saw him blow/below.
    I need a mint/minute to help me think.

The addition of semi-vowel y may be heard if you contrast the following:
    We tried to find the east/yeast.
    I earn/yearn a lot for the family.
    He had a good ear/year.

It would seem most useful to try and hear a clue from sounds that are impossible or confusing to lipread. For example, the shapes p, b, and m, are similar on the mouth but b is a voiced and louder sound and m is nasal in production and these differences might well be heard. Aware of this clue, the lipreader then has an auditory signal to help him distinguish similarities on the lips. Similarly, the suffix -ing is not a visible shape but may well be heard.
    Contrast the following:
    I'm tired of hearing about his pen/men.
    He's run up a bill/running up a bill.
    He found the rim/rib was broken.
    It's payday/May Day!
    Did you hear that crack/cracking?

It is common for listeners (and lipreaders) to transpose consonants: they will give lemon for melon, mane for name; this must happen in the mind.
    Try listening to these tranpositions: lisp lips, chanced chants, nest nets.

It is apparent that many of the lipreading exercises can be used as listening practice, just as listening practice material may be used for speech work. Each has its own particular problems and a teacher would emphasize different points, depending on the purpose of a lesson and the needs of the individual. A helper will recognize that the drills and repetitions used in the lipreading section can be utilized for listening sessions. All form part of the rehabilitative training that should be available to those with a hearing problem.

I have tried to make each section usable for lipreading (the essential), for listening practice (for those with residual hearing) and speech exercises (where the voice is deteriorating from its normal pattern). In practice sessions the situation is abnormal in that the helper is using written material and his delivery is likely to be slightly different from spontaneous speaking. I have tried to use colloquial forms wherever possible in order to simulate daily usage and would encourage the helper to change words which are not normally used by him or where a local dialect uses a different pronunciation. We teach sounds singly, that alter when in conjunction with others, that alter when said by different people, that alter when their position is changed, but the aim is to encourage a listening attitude and to develop the ability to recognize sounds correctly and speedily.

When the listener has begun to concentrate for longer spells then a more lengthy piece is possible. In the following piece the helper should write the words in capitals on slips that the listener can have before him and to which he can point as they appear in the text when it is read out to him.

I drove to Gatwick last weekend to meet a friend arriving by an afternoon plane from Italy.

As I reached the airport I saw the sign TERMINAL straight ahead.

A little further on I saw a SHORT TERM CAR PARK and left my car there.

I went past the sign saying ARRIVALS. I knew my friend would be coming through GATE 1.

Then I heard an announcement that her flight would be delayed BY TWO HOURS. I went back to THE MAIN

LOUNGE and strolled round the DUTY FREE SHOP. Then I took the escalator and went to THE COFFEE BAR on the first floor.

When my friend's plane landed she had some GOODS TO DECLARE. She also had to go to PASSPORT CONTROL so it was another two hours before we left Gatwick.

Mood in Speech

Listening to the mood of a voice is good practice, as is watching facial expression in lipreading. This material requires the helper to use first an *angry* tone of voice, so the delivery should be forceful and quite loud. Then the voice should hold a note of *enquiry*, there should be some hesitancy but no stridency.

To enable the listener to recognize the angry and enquiring tone, all the sentences in each block should be listened to at first. Then it is possible to select one or two from each to make selection more difficult.

Anger —   What does he think he's doing!
             That's the final straw!
             Just wait until I see him again!
             Who the devil does he think he is!
             I shan't stand much more of this!

Enquiry — Would you mind ringing my husband for me?
            Would you be so kind as to hold this for me please?
            Is this the right bus for Waterloo?
            Could you keep an eye on this for a moment please?

Intonation

In all countries people speak in different tunes. Chinese has a singsong effect; the Germans string a long collection of clauses and phrases together which end in a 'bang'; the Spanish give a lilting sound to their sentences. In English we use intonation to give meaning. When we make a statement we use a descending tone of voice, 'Her name was Mary Brown' When we ask a question the intonation starts high and descends, 'Where did that come from?'

However if we begin without an interrogative adverb or adjective (what, where, when, why etc.) the intonation will go up at the end, 'Were you planning to come?'.

When a statement is not complete the final stressed syllable slides upwards, 'Though we're all ready to go...' and it is important for the listener to note this change in intonation in order to decide whether a statement has been made, or an exclamation, or whether he has been asked a question.

It is useful to practise listening to the difference in stress and intonation in the following sentence pairs:

Do you come here *every* day?
Do you come *here* every day?
His arm was *broken*.
His *arm* was broken.
The nurse only broke her *wrist*.
The nurse only *broke* her wrist.
She always shops in *Oxford* Street.
She *always* shops in Oxford Street.

These are not always easy for the helper to do without practice but try to change your voice to say these in three ways, as a statement, as a question and then as an exclamation:

They didn't tell my father that.
They didn't tell my father that?
They didn't tell my father that!

Jones has scored.
Jones has scored?
Jones has scored!

Or take one sentence and try to accent each word in turn:

Would you like soup today?
Would *you* like soup today?
Would you *like* soup today?
Would you like *soup* today?
Would you like soup *today*?

Combining Sound and Vision

Although work has gone on in other countries for many years on the problems of adults with acquired hearing loss, and rehabilitative skills have been developed, little has been done in the UK to show how skills may be acquired using single sensory and bisensory methods of instruction. In 1977 a combined paper, issued by W.J. Watts and K.S.

Pegg, showed how a combination of visual and auditory channels reduced confusion. They showed that for many deafened adults the visual clues of lipreading did not provide enough information for efficient communication. Similarly, there were restrictions on the amount of auditory training which could be done to lead to a satisfactory level of speech discrimination. But by combining the two sensory channels each channel made some unique contribution to the intelligibility of speech which was not provided by either, singly. This investigation, which was funded by DHSS, pointed out that the most effective means of rehabilitation is one in which vision and hearing are combined to eliminate as much sensory confusion as possible. Such methods are available to few as yet, but a helper at home can go a long way to ploughing this furrow and giving practice to both senses singly and in combination.

On the telephone the deafened adult has problems with thirty/forty, which would not be so if he could see the speaker's face, since the shapes are dissimilar on the mouth. The following piece can be used both as lipreading and as listening drills:

It will take me thirty/forty minutes.

I think she's nearly thirty/forty.

Thirty/forty years ago it would not have mattered.

Now you owe me £30/£40.

The checkpoint in life is said to be forty.

At forty you should have tried to learn a musical instrument.

At forty you should have tried to learn a foreign language.

At forty you should have tried to travel to at least one foreign country.

At forty you should have tried to write a novel.

At forty you should have fallen in and out of love several times.

At forty you should have broken one or two bones.

At forty you should have learned to settle for much less than the ideal.

In the following sentences the number, thirty or forty, should be picked out:

There are thirty days in September.

Jesus was betrayed for thirty pieces of silver.

When Noah was in the Ark it rained for forty days and forty nights.
Jesus was in the wilderness for forty days.
There are thirty centimetres in one foot.

Involvement — a quick answer is required to these questions:
In which country would you be if
 — you were given forty marks in change?
 — picked thirty olives from a tree?
 — were forty feet up Snowdon?
 — paid thirty cents for a newspaper?
 — saw a herd of thirty elephants?
 — met a tribe of forty aborigines?
 — paid thirty francs for an ice cream?
 — saw thirty men leaning on their shovels?

The following short story is useful as listening or lipreading practice:
The Two Browns
There were two men named Brown. They were both fishermen and they lived in the same village. On the same day, one Brown lost his wife and the other Brown lost his boat.
The Vicar called on one of them, thinking it was the Brown who had lost his wife, but it wasn't.
The Vicar said to Brown, 'I am so sorry to hear of your loss.'
Brown replied, 'Oh, it doesn't matter. She wasn't up to much.'
'Indeed,' said the Vicar who was rather disgusted.
'No,' went on Brown, 'She was only an old thing. I offered her to a mate but he wouldn't have her. I've had my eye on another for a long time.'

In that story it is unlikely that the listener would hear the f and v sounds, although he may well guess the word from the context. If this doesn't happen then ask him to look and he will use his lipreading skill in conjunction with his hearing.

Useful drill: the helper needs to read the words through first aloud to himself so that a mistake is not made when reading the lines.

In each of these lines is a word that sounds different —
pick out the one with the different sound:

stone	telephone	shone	bone
clear	dear	near	wear
receive	dream	heard	seat
loop	fool	rule	door
rope	boar	soap	hope

Drill on nasals:

ever	never	every	everything
seven	eleven	seventy	heaven
clever	ever	heaven	seven

There seems nothing in this short drill — one line to be
used at a time — but the listener must be given the pattern
so many times for his mind to retain it in order to recall it.

After this, drill on the tens and teens is useful since this is
a lipreading problem that can be solved if the listener can
distinguish the nasal ending.

thirty thirteen, forty fourteen, fifty fifteen, and so on.

A similar dreary sounding exercise can be done to
emphasize the difference between a single and double
vowel, but I have never had a client say that he found the
practice boring. On the contrary he has been pleased to find
that he is able to learn the distinction.

Practise: bat/bite sat/sight pan/pine bat/bout Sal/soil

Here are two more intonation practices. The sympathetic
remarks should be made in a low quiet voice and the
disappointments make the voice descend at the end of the
sentence. Even if the listener cannot pick out all the words
of the sentence ask him to say whether he thought you
sounded sympathetic or disappointed.

Sympathy: I'm terribly sorry to hear the sad news.
You have all my sympathies, needless to
say.
Don't worry — you have a lot of good
friends to rally round you at this sad
time.
My dear, I'm so sorry.

Disappointment: I had such high hopes of him and now
look what's happened.

I don't think much of this dress now
I've bought it.
We worked so hard in the garden last
weekend and now look at what all that
rain has done to it.
Oh dear! I had hoped we could meet
before you went away.

A further example of using both a lipreading clue plus an aural one is in common words such as this/then/think/thank/that/though/thin/think. The person with the high frequency loss is unable to hear the sound of th but can lipread the shape that is made; yet it is likely that he will hear the nasal endings or/and the vowels of the above words.

Context is an additional guide as the following story shows — the listener should both watch and listen at first, and then repeat for listening practice alone.

The Insurance Man

An insurance man went to call on a newly married couple. The weather was cold and icy. The couple lived at the top of a steep hill so the insurance man was discouraged when the wife said that her husband was not at home. 'Where could I find him?' asked the insurance man. 'Well,' replied the wife, 'If he's where I think he is, fishing by the river, he could be in one of two places. If the ice is thick he'll be perched out *on* the river but if the ice is thin he'll be *in* the river.'

Now for practice on four other nasals — anything, nothing, something, everything:
There was an old woman
And nothing she had
Because she had nothing
They said she was mad.
She'd nothing to lose
She'd nothing to wear
She'd nothing to hope
She'd nothing to fear
She'd nothing to sell
She'd nothing to give
And when she did die
She'd nothing to leave.

Tell me anything you could do without.
Tell me something you would like to see changed.
Tell me everything you know about the Honey Bee.
Tell me something that is worth nothing.

Colloquial: He seems to know nothing about it.
He seems to know everything about it.
He seems to know something about it.
He seems not to know anything about it.

Now a few unconnected sentences to listen to stress — the listener should read the sentences first so that he knows what they are, he is concentrating on the rhythm of speech:
Somebody will find a use for it.
To *some* extent it works all right.
The nurse will look *after* you.
I'll see you in the *morning.*
The *sports* department may have them.
I suppose it's *reasonable.*

It is possible to show changes in rhythm and stress by building from a single word. For example, let the listener look at the following words and phrases:
in
in for
in form
in form at
in formation
information

Take care to make the last two sound different; then use the following sentences as build-up:
He was in.
He was in for a race.
He was in form for the race.
He was in form at the race meeting.
He was in formation on the parade ground.
He was seeking information. *Or* he was looking *for* in*for*mation (more difficult because of the repetition of for).

And:
in
in at
in at ten

inattention
He was in.
He was in at lunchtime.
He was in at ten for a coffee break.
He was punished for inattention.

Since many prefixes are unlipreadable try listening for a clue:
fined/confined
I was taken to the police station and I was fined/confined.
He is going to be fined/confined for the misdemeanour.

Conductor Joke
There was a bus conductor in America who pushed an old lady off his bus. The old lady died and the conductor was condemned to the electric chair. He was granted one request before the switch was pulled and he asked for a banana. When he had eaten the banana the switch was pulled but nothing happened. This was repeated twice more, so that after the third attempt the man had to be freed. Before he left prison the Governor said to him, 'I am curious. Was there something about those bananas that prevented the electricity from working?' 'Oh no,' the man replied, 'It's just that I am a bad conductor.'

To keep the listener's thoughts in one direction, ask him to listen and give you back the job or profession you have used in the following:
My firm wants another accountant.
My daughter is hoping to become a nurse.
At first she thought of being a secretary.
Her brother works as a travel agent.
He was going to be a policeman but changed his mind.
My wife was a buyer for a large firm before our marriage.
I started work as a freelance journalist. Later I became a reporter on one of the National newspapers. My hobby is gardening and I think I might have made a good nurseryman.

Back to *drill* — can you hear the difference between:
She was sopping/sobbing after her walk in the rain (one voiced, one unvoiced consonant) in all these examples.
He hit/hid his brother behind the house.

The fens/fence round our farm will keep trespassers away.
Is that badge/batch ready yet?
He wrote/rowed all morning.
He was carrying a rope/robe over his shoulders.
Will you get me a cab/cap please?

Differences between *vowels and stress*:
His tourists were injured. His two wrists were injured.
The queues at the hospital were heartrending. The cures at the hospital were heartening.
Did you see them Mary? Did you see them marry?
The horses legs were tied at night. The horses legs were tired at night.

The following is an extract which I read recently from the Lyttleton/Harte-Davis Letters. Lyttleton, who has become rather deaf says:

The National Health hearing aid is really unwearable — so clumsy and undiscriminating — you hear your own heart beating and, much louder than anything else, your own voice. My cynical Scotch friend said in answer to such complaints, 'Yes, I suspect half the hearing aids in England are put away in cupboards.'

Later on 5 October 1960:

Am trying a hearing aid which is modestly priced at £63. I hear with it everything I don't want to hear much more clearly, voices only a little. Last Sunday I wore it till the first hymn in which the organ, plus a handful of now stentorian voices, nearly blew me from my seat. On the whole I hate it, but whether I shall be brave enough to tell Mr Plume so on Saturday I gravely doubt. But £63!

And on 16 November 1960:

We called on the Cranworths yesterday. He has at 83 also taken to a hearing aid of the type that *my* good man said was *not* now satisfactory. He doesn't like it (Lord C) any more than I do mine but I handed on, to his comfort, the unanimous testimony to the good results of use and patience. At present if anyone drops a pin I am deafened by the din, but hear much less well the human voice. However, *my* comfort is that Pamela (his wife) definitely says she no longer has to bellow like a bull (wives do exaggerate you

know) at our tête-à-tête meals, so all is not lost. Poor old
Cranworth seemed to me to hear no better than before
(such was his belief too) but I fear that often his brain was
not taking it in.

To me the most important sentence there is the last — the
brain has to be able to make sense of signals fed in.

Of course hearing aids have improved greatly since those
days. Even so, many present wearers, because of their type
of loss and lack of training in its use, will recognize their
own reactions in much of what was said above.

If you possess residual hearing then, as regards speech
sounds, it is pertinent to listen for sounds of combinations
that may be invisible in lipreading. Prefixes are an example
— when truth looks like untruth and regular the same as
irregular, it is no wonder that the deaf make mistakes and
are thought stupid or contrary at times.

But often those little prefixes do contain a sound, such as
a nasal or a voiced consonant, that could be heard and
added to the lipread pattern.

Try listening to the following pairs of words and then
practise the repetition:

seat/*con*ceit — I'm glad I don't have his seat.
                — I'm glad I don't have his conceit.
                We are all full of small conceits.

Some of us are conceited about — the way we dress
Some of us are conceited about — our knowledge of a
     subject
Some of us are conceited about — our garden
Some of us are conceited about — the way we drive
Some of us are conceited about — the way we cook
Some of us are conceited about — the way we look
Some of us are conceited about — looking younger than
     our age
Some of us are conceited about — our knowledge of
     languages.

pose/*com*pose — I must try to pose myself for the
                   photograph.
                   I must try to compose myself for the
                   photograph.

meant/*com*ment — I wonder what he meant?
                   I wonder, what was his comment?

mute/*com*mute/*com*pute — (the last are two common words these days) —

Many people live outside a large town and have to commute to their work. G.K. Chesterton said, 'The only way of catching a train that I ever discovered is to miss the train before.'

If you are a commuter you spend a lot of time in travelling.

If you have a computer you save a lot of time unravelling.

Advertise presents difficulties to the lipreader as v is the first visible shape, which may well be thought of as f. Try listening to the word to see whether you find a clue in the voiced d (many people don't pronounce it) or do you hear the neutral a?

advert/advertise/advertising — listen to these several times over.

Samson had the right idea about advertising. He took two columns and brought down the house.

The oldest known advert was found in the ruins of Thebes in Greece. This offered payment for the return of a runaway slave.

The first advertisements in this country were in newspapers read in coffee houses, so that most of the first adverts were for coffee or tea. Now advertisements are all around us. We sleep on an advertised mattress, we get out of a bed that has been advertised, and we stand on an advertised carpet. In the bathroom we use an advertised soap and an advertised toothpaste.

There are secrets behind the glossy pictures of advertising. The steam from hot dishes is usually tobacco smoke because food tends to cool down too quickly for the photographer. Bubbles on soap are often Fairy Liquid because real bubbles burst too quickly. Whisky is substituted for tea because real tea has a scum on top and looks unattractive. And for beer advertisements sugar and egg white is stirred in to keep a good head on the glass. In fact advertising is the art of making you think you have longed for something all your life which you never heard of before!

The codfish lays 10,000 eggs

The homely hen lays one

The codfish never cackles
To tell you what she's done.
And so we scorn the codfish
While the humble hen we prize
Which only goes to show you
That it pays to advertise!

While we are mentioning advertising: do mention the fact that you have a hearing loss. Badges are available from the RNID and BAHOH indicating that you are a lipreader and would appreciate it if people spoke clearly to you. If you do not wish to wear a badge then inform the speaker so that he is aware of your problem. He needs information in order to help you, so words to the effect, 'I have a hearing loss — would you please speak a little slower and clearly for me' are useful to both sides.

Sound

Be aware of sound. Not only that, try always to identify what the sound is or what has made it. If you hear a bump — can you tell from which direction it came? Can you tell what caused it? If you hear a loud sound — was it inside or outside the house, was it someone talking? Try to pin it down.

Concentration is the key, as it is to a lipreading skill; let me illustrate by just one case how listening combined with lipreading proved useful.

Case History

Miss G. has a severe hearing loss in both ears, but because she has only a slight tailing off on the high frequencies she is still very much aware of sound. One would imagine that, with one or preferably two hearing aids, she could be brought up to a more meaningful level, in which case she would need training and adjusting to the new sounds since she has been receiving a much lower signal for the past four years. However, this lady has additional problems; a sensitive skin area and scalp damage following a very bad car crash. It has taken many many months for her to be able to tolerate any aid, for even a short length of time. Without the aid she hears sounds so softly that, given a word list, she finds it very difficult to distinguish sounds which fall closely together.

For example: for board she gives bird
    wall she gives wore
    vase   first
    them   then
    duck   dot
    boat   boot
    birth   bath
    car   for
    three   fast

Thus she has problems in deciphering long and short vowels, and she muddles nasals and voiced and unvoiced consonants. Lipreading helped her sort out some of these problems, but a lot of concentrated drill was needed on such phrases as:

Tomorrow is his bath/birthday. Come and listen to the bard/bird. The name/mane of that horse is black. It was my first yellow car/fast yellow car.

Using tapes of commonplace sounds, sounds made in the room we were using, and asking her to *say* words as well as *listen*, good progress was made. If Miss G. tries to lipread alone she is not very good; if she tries to listen without watching she understands nothing; but combining both signals she is able to understand extremely well.

The list on the next page can be used to discover whether the listener is mixing certain sounds, missing them entirely, or substituting. It can be useful for the helper to refer to from time to time or to use for short practice sessions.

Word Intelligibility Test
Take each section — say each word clearly and make a note of mistakes or substitutions.

warn	beam	shut	shawl
torn	bead	rut	ball
born	beach	but	squall
lawn	beak	nut	tall
meal	round	pearl	shirt
mill	bound	girl	dirt
mole	wound	whirl	flirt
mail	astound	curl	alert

He's vicious

He's superstitious

She's famous

She's aimless

She's amiable

He's hungry

He's angry

She's straight

She's strict

mushroom

workroom

bathroom

seep

seed

seethe

seek

daybreak

daylight

daytime

daydream

woodwork

woodworm

woodcraft

woodland

iceberg

icecream

icepack

northwest

northeast

northwind

hothouse

hotdog

hotfoot

hotcake

sidewalk

sidestep

playground

playtime

playroom

playmate

workshop

workroom

workhouse

7

SPEECH CONSERVATION

When I took the first survey of my undertaking, I found our
speech copious without order, and energetic without rules
Samuel Johnson

When Johnson wrote this preface to his great dictionary he
was referring to the problems of our language and since
language is conveyed most commonly through speech it
seemed an appropriate introduction to the problems of the
latter. I especially like the descriptions 'copious' and
'energetic', both of which so well indicate the richness of
our language.

I am using the word 'conservation' in preference to
'speech improvement' or 'correction'. Adults who suffer a
hearing loss have learned to speak naturally; this is not to
say that often some correction of badly pronounced words
or improvement of ill-made sounds would not come amiss
but means that they are not in the position of those who are
born without any ability to hear speech sounds and who
must learn to speak, which is a long, arduous struggle of
imitation and practice.

Speech is invulnerable to severe noise, distortion and
interference. We put our message into language form by
selecting the right words and phrases to express our
meaning and we place these in the correct order required
by the grammatical rules of our language. This process is
associated with activity in the speaker's brain and it is in the
brain that instructions are sent, by impulses along the motor
nerves, to move the muscles of the vocal organs, the
tongue, the lips and the vocal cords. It is these movements
which produce pressure changes in the surrounding air
known as sound waves.

In the speech chain there are really two listeners, not one, because the speaker listens to his own voice; this is known as feedback. Because we can hear ourselves we are able to control how loudly we speak, whether we are gabbling or speaking clearly and can make unconscious adjustments to produce the desired signals. Deafness deprives people of this speech feedback link. Even a slight loss can result in a loss of tone and a change in the speech pattern. A professional listener can, to some extent, tell the kind of deafness present from the type of speech deterioration it produces. In the very worst cases it is possible for the voice of a deafened adult to sound very much like the voice of someone who was born deaf.

To add to the problem of voice change is the fact that hearing people are often lazy listeners. If he has not really been concentrating or has been otherwise absorbed, a hearing person is often able to gauge what has been said by picking up just one or two clues, but if his ear picks up what he considers 'a strange sound' — possibly an unusual pitch or an odd flatness then his reaction is not even to try to decipher what is being said.

This presents the deaf adult with two tasks. First he must watch and lipread well enough to make sense of what is said to him and, secondly, he must take care to control his speech movements consciously and be aware of faults that can arise. To be able to perform both tasks adequately he needs instruction and someone with whom he can practise. He cannot lipread without having a partner to feed him conversation and he needs a good listener to pick out any speech fault and help to correct this.

To indicate that a person has poor speech can cause a violent reaction, not always from the deaf adult himself but from other members of the family, who have grown so used to a gradual deterioration that they are unaware of the need for tuition. It is normally the change in volume that is first noticed. An adult with a particular type of hearing loss will raise his voice considerably in an effort to hear his own voice. Another, who seems to hear his own voice very loudly, will start to speak in a whisper for fear he is shouting. Both of these results are socially unacceptable and usually cause some annoyance and irritation to the hearing members of a family.

I must emphasize that not all people with a hearing loss are going to become unintelligible and ostracized because of a change in their speech pattern. It is still not known why some people, despite a severe loss, have no more than a slight flatness in their voice even after decades of being deaf while others can show a voice change very rapidly, following a hearing loss. I have always tried to indicate gently, when a fault is evident, that some speech work would be beneficial — since communication is two-way then the listener must be able to know what you are saying without too great an effort on his part and it is often best to take the client individually, in order to work on the particular problems presented. Yet I also think group sessions can be an excellent source of speech conservation for adults who wish to maintain their good patterns and such classes have been amongst the most enjoyable I have taken.

Clients are often astonished at the intricate ways in which we use speech to denote meaning and become very interested in words and phrases, all of which, I maintain helps to promote their interest in lipreading. I know many deaf people — and of course there are hearing people in a similar position — who will not use certain words in our language because they have never heard them spoken. Of course they could consult a dictionary but this does not always help them to decide on a pronunciation. For example, I have a present client who will not use the word 'herpes', which has been much in the news recently, nor the word 'Xerox' because she has never heard them spoken, having been deaf since her teens. Once these are written down and the emphasis shown, and I explain that the X makes two different sounds in the last word, then I hope she might be confident to use them. I say might, because we all need to be sure of a word before we are happy about using it and this lady will be asked to practise the words many times before she gains enough confidence to trot them out unthinkingly.

I try to indicate that clear articulation is an asset worth acquiring. If the hard of hearing want hearing people to speak to them distinctly, they themselves must make an effort to be clearly understood. For a voice to be heard clearly and easily, there must be *vitality, projection and variety* in the speech act.

Vitality indicates the emotional quality of the voice, stemming from the thought behind the chosen words. This is often missing in speakers diffident about their views, those conscious of having poor speech, people in a depressed state or those trying very hard to make correct sounds. Some well-tried exercises on these points will be given at the end of this section.

Poor *projection* is the failure to control breath. Energy is lacking to send out sound waves to the listener in sufficient volume for him to hear them clearly. This lack of breath control accounts for the strangled, painful voices commonly heard in the hard of hearing circles. Incorrect use of breath and tongue results in nasality and poor tone.

Lack of *variety* is the failure to phrase speech and vary intonation and pitch, or the inability to use correct stress. These faults result in a monotonous voice, the assimilation of words, and a loss of word endings. Some or all of these faults may be present and it is important to maintain the good speech habits of the client or give therapy early before any bad habit can become fixed.

Giving therapy is the sticking point. It is common to rouse enthusiasm in a group of hard of hearing adults and then have to admit that they may well find it difficult to find a professional in their area who will carry out the necessary training. A Speech Therapist may be willing to consider someone with a hearing loss, although her list is likely to be long and priority will be given to stroke patients, stammerers and children with speech defects. A teacher of the deaf might be found to give evening lessons or a sympathetic Hearing Therapist might be able to give the necessary individual work. An elocutionist would be excellent, since singers have to produce a forward tone by using their facial cavities for resonance but this kind of help might prove expensive. There is no one discipline which can provide the speech work required by the hard of hearing under the National Health Scheme and this is a matter about which the British Association for the Hard of Hearing has been greatly concerned.

Recognition of the need for professional help is present but the professionals able to provide this are thin on the ground. The Health Service has been somewhat mean in its provisions for those who become deafened in later life.

Much spadework was required to begin the training of teachers of lipreading in this country — and these were considered to be needed on a part-time basis only, so that the shortest of courses was inaugurated. Until seven years ago there was no one professional body able to give the hard of hearing the necessary rehabilitation and no more than one dozen people are at present in training each year. Should anyone be unfortunate enough to lose a limb there is no delay in fitting a prosthesis and then instigating some therapy in order that that person may leave hospital able to use his false limb to the best of his ability. Certainly the deaf adult is issued with his prosthesis (the hearing aid) but advice on how and when to use this, the training required to combine its use with lipreading tuition, auditory training and, where necessary, speech work are largely unavailable over most of the country. This is a somewhat shortsighted policy since, if a one-legged man did not know how to use his new prosthesis or have practice in using it, then it would remain hidden in the wardrobe and, by the same precept, many hearing aids which are issued are left unused or not used to the full, indicating a great waste of time and money. If you live in a town then there is likely to be at least one lipreading class available but there is no register of a professional body of speech conservationists.

Teaching speech can be a problem. If the teacher shows any hesitancy or half-heartedness or is not wholly certain that it is a justifiable exercise, then this will communicate itself to the client. It is essential that the teacher performs first in order to promote the attitude 'this is essential, it is useful, we are doing this together and there is nobody else here to laugh at us'. Once this basic rapport has been established it is quite amazing what people are prepared to do — and it is not long before most will admit to enjoying the sessions very much. Much donkeywork is required in the early stages and it is essential that the class work be continued at home. For this reason it is helpful if a spouse or other relative can be shown the practice material and the points to be laboured, since the deaf adult will require a listener to monitor his attempts.

A point which often arises is the client's wish — 'I don't really want to talk "posh"'. This is a common misconception about speech conservation. It is not a matter of changing an accent or a dialect or sending people away able to mix in high society (since a number of upper-class accents leave much to be desired in regard to clarity this is not advisable anyway). The idea is to control the speech movements to prevent deterioration in enunciation; to understand what we actually do when we open our mouth to say a few words; to eliminate any unacceptable speech habits and to help clients become aware of faults which could arise should the hearing loss become greater.

The most common faults — and I hasten to add that these are not applicable solely to the hard of hearing — are as follows:

Nasality English is an acoustic language and the basic units of speech are distinctive sounds or phonemes. It is not a nasal language; very few of our sounds are made by the voice passing through the nose or more through the nose than the mouth. However, it is a common fault amongst the hard of hearing to pull the tongue back too far so that it blocks the passage of air through the mouth. It is helpful to feel the difference between a word with and without a nasal sound (e.g. mince/miss   tone/toe   nice/ice). If you are too deaf to hear yourself making a difference then it is easy to put one finger at the side of the bone in the nose and actually *feel* the difference.

A breathy voice This indicates a lack of breath control with more breath being used than the vocal chords can cope with. Slow and steady breathing exercises can help to expand the lower rib cage. Learning to blow a candle flame so that the flame is bent but does not go out, or sustaining vowels without the flame flickering teaches control. No adult is likely to do such antics without seeing the teacher demonstrating both the method and result.

A throaty or gutteral voice would require much exercise on forward vowels since the voice is being produced too far back because of retraction of tongue.

Jerky utterance indicates faulty breath control. Exercises progressing to reading and conversation are helpful.

A flat toneless voice is common in cases of severe and long-standing deafness — there is lack of rhythm and accent and little expression. This is a very important point since we use pitch in speech actually to change meaning. Take a phrase such as 'Smith has scored' as an example. Without inflection it is a statement. With a rise in pitch it becomes a question — 'Smith has scored?' And with greater energy and different emphasis it will become an exclamation — 'Smith has scored!'

We alter the pitch of our voice to denote the emotions we feel. A low, quiet voice to say 'I'm terribly sorry to hear the sad news' would show our sympathy while a more energetic, quicker voice to say 'I've had a terrific time this weekend' would help the listener experience some of our enthusiasm. In speech work it is interesting to see how many hard of hearing people find this difficult and need much practical work to put emotion into their words.

A high pitched voice is often the result of a low tone loss. It is possible to find by trial the speaker's vowel which is nearest to normal pitch (there is usually at least one) and then tune the others to it.

Failing to sound consonants indicates a lazy tongue and lip action. Leaving off the final consonants in a word or swallowing these results in speech that is difficult for a listener to follow, since sentences become a series of vowels only. This is one of the easiest faults to correct with exercises on short words that keep the tongue moving and in correct position.

Drawling may sound like a whine and give a false impression of the speaker's personality. There is vocalizing of nearly all the elements of speech and a linking of the last sound in one word with the beginning of the next. It is possible to correct by splitting the elements of a phrase, using touch on throat to detect when voice is present. There needs to be a complete break between each word to start with but the interval can be shortened to a normal rate of speech as soon as it can be done without drawling.

One of the great difficulties for an adult who cannot hear his own speech at all is to know when he is using voice and when he is not. It is possible to speak voicelessly — in fact many of our consonants are made correctly in this way.

Since we do not actually know very much about the origins of speech I like to think that the first sounds were probably the loud shouts of a good strong voice, using the vocal cords. Then, as the brain developed and we needed more language to express ourselves we found we needed more sounds to express this language and one refined way in which to do this was to make a speech movement that we already knew but this time without vibrating the vocal apparatus. For example, a p is the unvoiced version of the sound b and an f that of the voiced v. Children who are born severely deaf have to conquer this problem with visual and kinaesthetic aids but it is difficult to find an ideal voice vibrator that would assist the hard of hearing adult. A prototype was tried out by the RNID in 1978 which would give a vibration signal for the voice level of the wearer and, to a limited extent, of other voices and sounds in the vicinity. However, the aid was a finger attachment that was rather delicate and easily damaged so that although initial response was excellent, practically it was not found suitable. One psychological point was that the prototype did seem to reduce some of the deafness frustration in the more withdrawn testers but the experimenters were surprised to find that there were some deaf people who did not respond to the vibration at all.

It is my experience that there is indeed a wide variation in response to vibration and, during the latter years of teaching, I have met adults who have seemed 'dead' to all forms of conducted sound. In some cases these adults have lost all hearing after large doses of drugs required to cure a severe illness or given following a kidney transplant. They had no real option but to take the dosage, which left them without sound but with severe tinnitus. When two women with this problem underwent tests, neither could detect any vibration of a ringing telephone when placing their hands on the receiver and one of them failed to detect anything when her husband thumped on the piano and she stood behind with her hands on the instrument. Both have responded, during speech work, to the feel of their speech on jaw, nose, throat and chest and a vibrator which could be worn at the throat would possibly have proved useful.

There are indeed limitations on the changing of fixed speech patterns and habits. It is said to be impossible to introduce modulation into a 'deaf' voice but, even here, emphasis can be tried which will give the impression of some rise and fall in the voice. Stressing different words in a sentence is useful practice:

"Did you catch the *plane?*" (not the train or the bus)
"Did you *catch* the plane?" (not miss it)
He's going to look after the *baby*. (not the dog)
He's going to look after the baby. (his wife is not)

Stress is an important part of speech work because we change emphasis in English to make one part of speech different from another. Words with two or more syllables exhibit distinctive patterns of accent associated with pitch and stress.

a*tt*ribute (noun)   *e*nvelope (noun)   *permit* (noun)
attr*i*bute (verb)   env*e*lope (verb)   perm*i*t (verb)

You can hear that these are quite small changes requiring a difference in length of vowel and stress. I can remember a story in one of Ellery Queen's Crime Wave novels in which a murder mystery was based on word puzzles and the fact that the same word may mean different things to different men, working in different fields. The argument arose about the word UNIONIZED. Most of the men in the party stressed the first syllable, pronouncing it as YOO-NIONIZED but the two scientists present read it as UN-EYE-ONIZED and this illustrates the fact that no two people have exactly the same language. Fortunately there is sufficient overlap for us to understand each other but with new words and phrases added to our language every day, the hard of hearing may well miss out on adding these to their vocabulary.

Speech does need to be precise to be accurate in meaning. English depends on this for its finer nuances. If the tongue is indecisive or slips, then alternate meanings are made. Try to say the following phrases quickly and still keep each word distinct and you will find it is not so easy unless you make yourself slow down just a little.

He's discussed it with me.   He's disgusted with me.
We talked about pastimes.   We talked about past times.
That's a good answer.   That's a good dancer.
I'll give them that before tea.   I'll give them that beef for tea.

Think of the small differences between:

the world of tomorrow/the whirl of tomorrow
When do you leave?/Where do you live?

In rapid speech the sounds are bound to be equivocal.
How often do we say: Jew know him?

It's alright frim.
Let's go out fra bit.
What major do it?
He's got it infamy.
He fell office horse.
I've rapture parcels.

even   Ammonia little one.

Of course we understand these and it is this sort of speech that makes our language so rich in word jokes, like the following:

A man said to a fairy, 'Do fairies have names?'
'Yes,' said the fairy, 'my name is Nuff.'
'I've never heard of that name before,' said the man.
The fairy replied, 'Surely everyone has heard of Fairy Nuff?'

Sometimes, well knowing that we are going to have difficulties, we will alter our words in order to overcome a foreseeable difficulty — rather than attempt 'I'll wait in the foyer for her' we might more easily say 'I'll wait here for her.' But if we could be more precise in making the sounds of the words we use then this clarity would be of the greatest benefit to the lipreader and perhaps we would take a greater pride in listening to the interesting language which is ours to speak as we will.

As with lipreading, there must always be a realistic goal in speech work. Limitations are the impossibility of introducing normal modulation in a 'deaf' voice; the unlikelihood of changing some fixed speech patterns and habits, and the capacity of the client to give sufficient time and interest. The greatest hopes are in creating a 'thinking' speech habit; to monitor speed so that slowing down enables final consonants to be made properly, and controlling volume and improving breath control. To attain just one of these goals will achieve some improvement. I have found that the most rapid advances have been where a deaf and a hearing person can attend a class together and also be prepared to practise exercises between teaching sessions. If the deaf adult has been referred for lipreading but is also prepared to spend part of a session in speech practice, then he is usually much more concerned about the former. He sees lipreading as the only way to maintain normal communication and this is his first priority. In some cases, where it is imperative that he work at speech, the deaf adult may still find it difficult to accept the need simply because he cannot hear his mistakes. Then the hearing helper is of tremendous help in confirming that the need is there. It is possible to give simple breath control exercises to be done at home daily, exercises to keep the voice forward in the mouth and others for tongue and lips or better enunciation. The instructor should, of course, deal with any individual faults during the teaching session and the final chapters will include material which has been found useful and enjoyable as well as a suggested scheme that can be worked through, or tailored to a client's needs.

A good teacher of speech must first learn to listen and diagnose and the following suggestions may prove helpful. A client needs to be told that you are going to spend some time listening while he talks to enable you to pick out any faults requiring attention. Some clients will say what they consider is wrong with their speech, often mentioning one specific point such as 'I can't make a proper F'. Asking them to read aloud will give an indication of some faults but, wherever possible, it is better to carry on a conversation and hear the natural voice. Try to take note of:

Speed — is this too fast, too slow, too hesitant?
Pitch — is the voice pitched too high, too low or is there lack of modulatory control?
Intensity — is the volume too loud, too soft, too variable (going from loud to soft uncontrollably)?
Tone — is the voice harsh, gutteral, too nasal, too thin?
Word-endings — are these lacking, swallowed, slurred, merged into the following word?
Sound distortions — is the client making incorrect vowels? (Remember he may now be hearing these distortedly.) Making ur for or is a common error; the consonants w, l and r are sometimes made incorrectly or interchanged

and there are many difficulties with double and treble consonants.

It is not possible, in one session, to diagnose all faults. It is better to make a note, during the first weeks, of all errors; and then concentrate on those most sociably unacceptable — that is, pitch, volume and the word-endings.

As in any skill, little is learned at any one time and although a variety of material might be used to maintain interest and incentive, insight must be kept the main aim of each particular client. If breathing is poor, then this fact must be stressed throughout; if enunciation requires polish, then this is the constant reminder; if volume is to be controlled, then this must be emphasized throughout each part of the lesson at every meeting. Few of us think of what we are doing when we speak as it is a function which we expect to continue naturally. In the anxious early days when a client knows his own voice sounds 'different' — sometimes this is only because he has to accustom himself to hearing his own speech through an aid and may sound perfectly natural to the listener — it is then possible to begin to interest him in the miracle of speech. He has to be convinced first that there is every probability that as his hearing loss progresses then some deterioration in his voice will become apparent. He has to realize that, to the public, this would be more off-putting than any inability to lipread and that work in the early stages will maintain a good speech pattern. A few fascinating facts and a little preliminary exercise usually convinces him that 'there is something in this'. Some of the initial points I try to make are:

Clenched teeth will not make for good or clear speech. Hold the back of your hand half an inch or so under your jaw and say 'far, far away'. Did your jaw touch your hand? If so, how many times? And if not, then you are afraid to open your mouth to let the sound come out.

Monotony of voice makes listening more difficult and sleep more attractive. Monotony is often caused because the voice is all on one note and has no change of tone. Try this exercise with me; say 12345 first making your voice go up the scale (do not sing, just use your speaking voice). Then go down the scale. Still saying 12345 make it sound like a question — an invitation — a refusal — say it to express anger — in sorrow — in joy — simply by changing the tone and inflection of your voice.

Circumstances will alter your way of speaking. Learn to be adaptable and flexible. It is no use speaking to a group in a large room with the same amount of voice that you would use for an intimate chat to a friend at your side. If you speak in an ordinary conversational voice in a large room then only the front row will hear you. Time has to be allowed for sound to travel. Voice is quickly lost once it leaves the mouth and so it must be projected. You can learn to read a piece as though you were telling a bedtime story; then again as you would speak in your sitting room and yet again to be heard in a big hall. All this practice will give you control of your voice.

For breath control. Take a deep breath, count to 20 — let out any remaining air. Now try 25 then 30.

Take a deep breath. Hold one nostril closed and count to 5 in your head, then hold both closed and count another 5, let one nostril go free and count another 5, let the other go and see if you have any breath left. If you have, then try counting to 7, then 9.

Take in breath quickly through the mouth and then let it escape in a hiss. Relax, repeat, always letting the breath escape evenly.

Now use your lips and breath. Breathe in, then breathe out slowly whispering 'one, two, three'. Don't use your voice, the words are formed by the lips alone. Do this several times. Repeat, whispering up to 8 in an even stream as you breathe out.

To keep your voice forward
Hum . . . Can you feel your lips vibrating? Check by slightly parting and closing lips and feel the vibration as you say mumm mumm mumm.
Say the sound of ah (as in far) and you will notice your jaw move downwards.
Now say ah again and pinch your nose. There should be *no* difference in the sound when your nose is pinched or unpinched.

Stimulate the ear of the listener. Try saying the following,
stressing a different word each time:
Would you like soup *today?*
Would you like *soup* today?
Would you *like* soup today?
Would *you* like soup today?
Would you like soup today?
You just don't know what we've been *through.*
You just don't *know* what we've been through.

'We're going to Margate again for our holidays' — say this in
a happy tone of voice, then in a miserable tone of voice,
then in an exasperated tone, then in an angry tone. In other
words, make your voice act your words.

You may well imagine that no one is going to dash merrily
into this work without someone to act as example and give
encouragement — an enthusiastic and congenial teacher is
imperative. Although the following sections are related to a
teaching programme and are, therefore, more pertinent to
teachers and teaching material, they are meant to be useful
to those who are unable to attend a class or who are able to
work with a helper at home. Few teaching tools are
required. It is helpful to have a mirror to hand; a pack of
tissues to mop the dribbles when the tongue becomes
overwrought, and a drink for lubrication. If a teacher has a
Linco aid, sound level meter and vibrator available then
these are indeed useful aids but a good listener is more
essential.

It is not necessary to have a knowledge of phonetics to
carry out useful speech conservation. Phonetics is the
science of speech. You may remember Eliza Doolittle
saying 'That ain't proper writing' when Professor Higgins
wrote down her speech sounds but our purpose is a little
more humble, we merely want to understand the elements
of speech. We want to understand phonology which is the
way that speech sounds relate to their linguistic function.
An example will make this clear: 'cool', 'kill' and 'keel' all
begin with the k sound. If you listen carefully you will hear
that they are not exactly alike. They are all recognizably k
sounds but in *cool* the k is made a little further back in the
mouth. The k in *keel* is nearer the teeth than it is in *kill*. So

there is a general class of k sound called the family or phoneme. The types of sound within the family are called allophones. Try with other words such as 'ten', 'tea' and 'tar' and you will find the same thing applies to the t.

To the phonetician these divisions are of great interest — it is his joy to note scientifically every single possible human sound — but the phonologist is concerned mainly with the semantics or meaning of sounds.

However, whichever branch of sound we are interested in — the scientific or linguistic — we have to have a means of notating the sounds. The roman alphabet is not large enough because one letter can make more than one sound e.g. 'A' may be pronounced differently depending whether you are saying path or age or apple. Therefore symbols have been devised by the International Phonetic Association and these often puzzle a speaker when he resorts to a book on Speech Therapy for practice material. For the client willing to learn these symbols and able to apply them the system is excellent but most laymen would prefer not to and then finding material is difficult. Whatever material is used it *is* important for the client to consider the Organs of Speech in a non-technical way.

Speech sounds are made out of out-breathed air. This we all appreciate. The air is moulded into different shapes, obstructed and then released, or allowed to escape under pressure by the use of the tongue, lips, teeth and jaw movements. For example,

we can make the sound oo by moulding our lips and letting the air come through the shape we have made;

we can make the sound p by keeping our lips together, holding the breath inside and then suddenly opening the lips so that the air explodes and creates sound;

we can make the sound f by resting our top teeth on our lower lip, holding the air then allowing it to escape by pushing it through the gaps.

What experimenting must have taken place at the

beginnings of recognized speech!

Most languages make speech from out-breathed air although some African languages use an in-breathed or imploded sound at the start of some words. In such a name as Mboya the speaker starts with an inbreathed m. In the upper part of the windpipe lies the larynx (Adam's apple) which holds and protects the vocal cords. These are like a pair of lips that stretch across the larynx from front to back; they are tough pieces of membrane which come together and separate. The space between is the glottis — which is the Greek word for voice — but it is the cords themselves which constitute the voice. Air makes them vibrate and it is this which gives the musical sound we hear in song. One assumes that the first meaningful sounds were all made with voice and, later, when it was found that there were few other movements we could make with our mouths and tongue, then we stopped moving our vocal cords to produce other letters. This has led to difficulties for the lipreader who is unable to judge when the vocal cords have been vibrated but it has been a means of increasing sounds and language. Yet the vibration is not enough to provide richness and we need resonators to magnify the sound produced by the voice. These are provided by the chest, throat, mouth and nasal cavities and this underlines the need for breathing exercises and for taking care of our general health so that our sinuses and nasal passages are clear and thus able to act as magnifiers. There would not be much speech without the voice; people whose vocal cords have been destroyed by throat cancer, or sufferers from bad attacks of laryngitis, have to find a substitute by sending air up from the stomach or be equipped with an artificial larynx in order to be heard.

A speech sound disappears in twelve seconds, so is soon lost if there is no energy behind it and research has shown that only 45 per cent of the public use a voice over a sixty decibel level — in other words their voice would not carry very far nor be heard clearly by anyone with a hearing loss, so that unless a speaker has a clear, strong voice the deaf adult is deprived of essential aural clues. Speech and the ways in which we can use (or abuse) our voice are worth a study and I would hope that the material given at the end of this book will encourage both deafened adult and the helper to enjoy the work more.

If you have a hearing loss, you will keep on watching for visual clues and you will, if you wear an aid and have residual hearing, listen intently. Now I will consider the third aspect of a hearing loss — the possible loss of normal speech pattern and clarity. I say 'possible' because it would be incorrect to say that all deafened adults lose control over their speech to the extent that it becomes almost unintelligible; but with any loss there is a change of tone and often a flattening and change of pitch. Much depends on the degree of hearing loss for speech tones.

It is an incredible fact that when an adult, who has used speech for most of his life, is suddenly deafened and no longer able to hear his own voice, he loses control of the 'music' of his voice. He has lost the feedback through his own ears, which has enabled him to monitor his speech and to correct it if necessary. And it may be the last straw to learn that, as well as needing to step up visual and aural attention, he also needs to be aware of his speech pattern. Lipreaders can pretend, they can smile and nod and appear to understand, but speak with an unnatural tone or in a 'deaf' voice and members of the public will often not bother to try to decipher what is said. Professional help is available to few and there needs to be sympathy and a lack of hesitancy on the part of any helper if speech practice at home is to prove worthwhile. Yet it can be fun — rhythm is enjoyable and good speech is a pleasure — and speaking out loud is excellent oiling for the vocal cords.

So I would suggest you approach the practice exercises with a view to enjoying the sound of your voice, being precise where clarity is essential, and gaining as much pleasure from the swing and measure of words as is possible from music.

In some exercises it is possible to aid the helper by pointing out the importance of certain sounds but in other cases instruction would need to be long and technical. As stated, professional tuition is vital in some cases, and should always be sought when a voice change is noticeable but, as I have been able to confirm in classes, conservation is possible if attention is paid to the voice and some short practical sessions undertaken.

An adult feels self-conscious and foolish boo-ing and baa-ing before an audience — I had one client who would go to the bottom of his garden for the vocal exercises `— yet professional singers need to do these all the time to maintain good voice and we all carol at some point in our bathrooms.

Speech Conservation Programme

You should pass over this section if, as a helper, you feel that this is too technical. But the following programme has proved useful.

The adult, although he has no need to be taught speech sounds as is necessary with a born deaf child, nor a mode of delivery as with a stammerer, nevertheless has probably given little thought all his life to speech production. Clients have been interested to realize what a miracle speech is, how precise movements need to be within the small confines of a mouth, as well as the fun that can be had from the stress and rhythm of words and phrases.

As a teacher, a progressive syllabus is always necessary and the following is one that takes difficulties step by step.

1. A talk on *delivery*: that there must be *thought* before speech;

   that *phrasing* is determined by meaning — have practice pieces ready phrased; try to manage breathing so that no pause for breath breaks the continuity of the phrase. Make slight pauses at the end of the phrases.

   show that *emphasis* is not only correct stress but also part of personality;

   show that *rhythm* helps to retain and maintain meaning;

   show that *intonation* is the variety of pitch — naturally; acquired from local dialect or the family voice and a tone change indicates emotion.

Practise

Don't do that again! (Express anger/fear/deprecation/expostulation.)

This is just what I expected! (Delight/anger/despair.)

So, this is what you tried to tell me about. (Delighted surprise/anger/disappointment.)

Did you know about this before you invited me? (Interest, reproach, pleasure, shame.)

2. *Mastery of sounds in words*, then phrases, excluding complex or difficult sound combinations.
   E.g. t as in take, matter, met, tearitup,
   but *not* tray, mostly, acts, about the house... (these involve combinations of two or more consonants).

3. *Combinations of 2 consonants*
   E.g. gl as in glass, ugly, 'The bagleaks at the end', and 1m as in almanac, elm, 'It took me almost allmorning', and pb as in soapbag, 'Leapback before you get splashed'.

4. *3 or more consonants:* English, explain, luncheon, handled.

5. *Closely related vowels:* food, foot, net, knit.

6. *Reading exercises:* to fix (entrench) improved speech habits.
   Useful material would be a good mixture of literary selections, jingles, limericks, dramatic readings.

7. *Special combinations of 2 consonants* relating to *pressure elements*, for example getting to a fricative from a plosive, as in thick veil.
   And *voiceless/voiced consonants:* keep Bob's knife,
   cut Beryl's hair

The closer the physiological adjustments for 2 consonants, the more difficult it is to say these, as an example the word 'lisp' is easy because s and p are involved with different articulators, but the word 'test' is difficult because s and t are close to each other.

8. *The vowel murmur* in such words as:
   about, moment, possess, volunteer, porous, vanity, porpoise, Dinah, and righteous.

In many words we do not articulate the correct vowel but substitute the murmur. It does not appear in lipreading yet it is most commonly used and is important in securing the rhythm of speech.
   It is worth both trying to lipread a difference and hear a difference between sentences like the following,
   Can he ford/afford the river running through his property?
   Give way/Give away.
   Live/liver.

Articulatory Phonetics

Let us now return to exercises we can all profitably do, after a few preliminaries on what are called articulatory phonetics, i.e. the function of speech through correct production by the movement and position of the vocal organs. Anything we say can be fairly well described as having three strands — the rhythm of the sentence, the melody, and the individual speech sounds themselves. When we talk we use certain organs of the body, because most sounds are made by causing air to move either through the mouth, or through the nose, or through both. The lips and the cheeks influence speech in more than one way. They change the shape of the vocal tract and, consequently, the kind of speech sound produced. Together with the teeth, they are the only parts of the vocal tract normally visible. The teeth are used to restrict or stop the flow of air either by placing them close to the lips or the tip of the tongue. The tongue and the lips also play a part, so that any exercises we can give to improve voice production must involve all of these organs.

Exercises for Lips

The muscles controlling the lips are on the face — at the rim of the eye sockets, the cheekbones just at the ears, and the angles of chin — so that lip movements involve the whole surface of the cheeks. Failing to use the lips will result in a mumble. Another fault, amongst women in particular, is to use a backward stretch of the corners of the lips consistently. It is a characteristic of the too highly strung and results in a thin, hard timbre.

For good voice production the lips must alternate between natural posture. (stretching back only for s and z and vowels i/e) and the rounded position as for w, oo, o, u.

Try: 1. Press lips firmly together then release.
     2. Smile/pout, keep centre of lips free from teeth.
     3. Alternate between vowels — i-oo, u-i, e-o, o-ee.

Exercises for the Tongue

The tongue is normally relaxed for breathing. The portion behind the teeth is broad and flat. When no point is used in this relaxed position then we hear the thick, indistinct articulation and the lalling common in the mental defective, but varying degrees of this are at the root of most bad speech.

Good voice production requires skilfully adjusted tongue movement. The muscles must be flexible in order to have a firm, round point. This is unconsciously achieved when a person lives in an atmosphere of cultured speech, imitating good voices from childhood. When someone is used to a mumbled, slovenly speech, specific tongue training is required. Stiffness must be avoided — this produces faulty resonance and throatiness.

Keep the tongue flat and keep saying *ah*, trying to go up three notes — *ah, ah, ah*.

For very stiff tongues place the end of tongue on lower lip then stretch tongue out and up without touching the lips — this stretches the fraenum, the bridge of tissue under the tongue.

Breathing Exercises
By now the purists will be taking issue with me for not having stressed breathing exercises — the basis of all speech production. This is because I have found clients most reluctant to perform these on their own. However, breath is the vehicle of voice so here are exercises for breath control that you *should* do every day.

1. Breathe in through the nose and out through the mouth slowly and steadily. If you rest your hands lightly on your lower ribs you should feel expansion sideways when you breathe in and contraction as you breathe out. Do you? Many people will not find this at first because they are breathing up and down, rather than letting the ribs expand sideways.
2. Take in breath quickly through the mouth and then let it escape in an even hiss. Relax and repeat.
3. Breathe in. Breathe out slowly, whispering 1-2-3. Don't use voice, the words are formed by lips alone. Relax. Do this exercise several times. Repeat, whispering up to 8 in an even stream as you breathe out.
Your voice should not be swallowed, keep it forward.
4. Repeat numbers 1–5 and imagine you are saying these to someone in a far corner — OVER THERE!

Now try another exercise to aid clear articulation.

You would imagine that adults would balk at blowing bits of tissue about, but I have always found it an effective and accepted means to make a point. Place some bits of tissue on the back of your hand. Then say, 'Pay the piper'. Each time you articulate the sound of p you should make a little explosion of breath so that bits of paper fly off your hand. Now try again with the sound t (remember to make it as ta and not tee). The word 'titter' should scatter your paper twice. Hold your hand near your lips and as you say, 'Cut the cake' feel the draught on your hand every time k is sounded; now try saying 'Be kind to cats' or, 'The call of the cuckoo'.

In such ways adults will realize the importance that breath and articulation have in speech. They know they have to open their mouths, since the sound cannot come out otherwise, but they have never needed to question how and what they are doing inside the mouth each time they make an utterance.

We will first attempt a few prose pieces and set pieces for clear speech. I have indicated the most obvious difficulties so that a helper will know what to listen for; it is best to allow the reader to go through the piece without interruption, after he has had time to absorb the sense, and then point out any sound combinations that were not distinct. Since these are not conversational pieces, they should be read at a steady pace and each word given its true sound so that it would be heard perfectly by any audience.

Tonight we are very fortunate to have Professor Higgins to speak to us. The Professor is an expert on flowers — particularly those that grow in mountainous regions — and he has chosen 'The Flowers of Snowdonia' for his talk tonight. This he will illustrate by a series of slides that he has brought with him, so I am sure we shall all spend a most enjoyable and instructive evening. I ask you all to welcome — Professor Higgins!

Difficulties:
to speak to us — k should be clear and phrasing correct,
expert — eks not eggs-pert,
particularly — five syllables to enunciate,
illustrated — 3 consonants, str,

series of slides — sibilants must be clear not slushy,
shall all spend — clear vowels required,
instructive evening — two vs must be made.

By doing a good deal of this type of practice a client was given sufficient confidence to stand and make similar introductions at his local club meetings. The main faults are usually too rapid speech, falling voice at end of sentences, and insufficient stress. The helper must remember that only one point can be expected to be improved in each session. If you are concentrating on diction then do not pick on other faults, or the reader becomes overwhelmed at all he must remember.
    Try the next piece.

This will be our sixteenth annual Jumble Sale since our Club started in 1969. Each year we seem to accumulate more jumble, more willing helpers, and provide more stalls. Let us hope that we shall also make more money! If you are able to volunteer to man a stall, help with the collections, or just give an hour of your time, then please give your name to Mrs Harris before you leave tonight. Thank you.

Difficulties:
16th/1969 — numbers must be clear and stressed,
each year — ch must be clear and not sh (neither should it
    sound like cheer),
accumulate — all syllables sounded,
emphasis on *more* each time,
to man a stall — each word distinct — not manner stall,
collections — two ks,
give an hour — each word distinct, not anour,
Harris — no over-breathed h.

Now here is a piece for final consonants, t/k/n. Since t and n are the most common finals they are obviously worth a practice.

Afternoon tea is a curious meal. In England, the land of its birth, it is without honour; people drink it standing up, sitting down, or walking about — at a table, at a desk, or off the corner of the mantelpiece; sometimes it is merely imbibed from a Thermos flask in the back office. No Englishman or Scotsman really cares where or how he has his tea, as long as he gets it. Foreigners have missed the point of tea, which is that it is above all things a hugger-mugger affair.

Difficulties
On first glance this appears simple, but to give each word its weight and to stress the piece sensibly is a little more complicated. Phrases such as drink it, walking about, at a table, or off the, back office, he has his, he gets it, that it is above all, should all be practised in isolation before a second read.

The next piece combines intonation with emotive sound. There are so many adjectives for colour or jewels that it is a good piece for stressing important words and for correct breathing — you will see that a pause or breath needs to be taken between the colour and name of the jewel for the piece to make sense.

He came back down from the terrace and stopped in the garden to look at the fruit. The trees in this garden were all laden with the most extraordinary fruit. The fruit of each tree had a separate colour. Some were white, others green, blue or violet and some of a yellowish hue. The white globes were pearls; the sparkling and transparent fruits were diamonds; the deep reds were rubies, the green, emeralds; the blue, sapphires; the violet, amethysts; those tinged with yellow, topaz. Aladdin was not yet of an age to be acquainted with the value of these stones and he thought they were only pieces of coloured glass.

The next piece is rather different and not so easy to manipulate. It is a sermon ascribed to Muhammed but it is so like many of the repetitive stories told to children that it possibly formed the basis for these. The questions mean keeping the voice up at the end of the sentences and one long sentence towards the end means having enough breath that the reader does not gasp his way through.

When God made the Earth it shook to and fro till He put mountains on it to keep it firm.
    Then the Angels asked, 'O God, is there anything in thy creation stronger than these mountains?'
    And God replied, 'Iron is stronger than the mountains, for it breaks them.'

'And is there anything in thy creation stronger than iron?'

'Yes, fire is stronger than iron for it melts it.'

'Is there anything stronger than fire?'

'Yes, water for it quenches fire.'

'Is there anything stronger than water?'

'Yes, wind for it puts water in motion.'

'Is there anything stronger than the wind?'

'Yes, a good man giving alms.'

'If he gives it with his right hand and conceals it from his left, he overcomes all things.'

'Every good act is charity.'

'Your smiling in your brother's face, your putting a wanderer on the right road, your giving water to the thirsty is charity.'

'A man's true wealth hereafter is the good he has done to his fellow men.'

'When he dies people will ask what property has he left behind him?'

'But the Angels will ask, "What good deeds has he sent before him?" '

PART TWO

LIPREADING PRACTICE

It is a person's attitude towards his handicap that ultimately determines the real seriousness of it. The way he views his handicap is important. A healthy approach would be to take it on the chin, don't run away from it, and don't fight it. Viewing it objectively is not easy but is more positive than a deep emotional reaction.

The more intelligently clients have dealt with their handicap, the better their adjustment. None of which is to decry the fact that deafness is a crippling handicap, little understood by the majority of the public and some professionals.

I view with suspicion the belief that suffering ennobles the character. I am sure that if a man was an unlikeable character before his deafness he will continue to be an unlikeable character after deafness has struck. William James said that, 'a difference is only a difference when it makes a difference' and some people let their ears make a difference and over-estimate the number of closed doors. A person is surely more than his ears, and it behoves any willing helper or teacher to give advice and practical help that will enable deafened adults to use what senses they retain, any hearing they still possess and learn a new skill to the limit of their capacity to enable them to prise doors open again. I believe people can do this only if they become expert on their own hearing loss.

So now on with the lipreading practice.

A Summary
Those who have to lipread — and this means anyone with even a slight loss — are using a skill which, like any other

skill, may be picked up naturally to some extent but which will improve with good tuition and practice.

Lipreading is dependent first on the *eye* — if the eye cannot catch the shape of the words then no information is available.

Suggestions — to the speaker: slow your rate of utterance but try not to change the rhythm of speech;

Watch yourself say 'Good morning, how are you?' quickly and then slow it up *too* much and see the change in pattern;

Turn down your television set and see how much *you* understand when you see lip movements only;

Try to imagine how long you would be able to concentrate if you had to lipread all day.

Suggestions — to the deafened: Try to do exercises to improve your speed of lipreading;

Try to concentrate a little longer each day;

Give your eyes a rest when you are alone;

Watch for the *rhythm* of speech and don't try to catch or analyse each word.

The *eye* is helped out by the *ear* — this is not the case if the deaf person is very severely deaf, and no longer hears sound, but most deafened adults have some useful residual hearing that can be trained to help the eye.

Suggestions — to the speaker: Do not shout but try to use a strong, clear voice;

Speak into the hearing aid if the listener is wearing a body-worn aid, asking him to hold it between you;

Try to give a clue, e.g. stress the important word in your conversation — perhaps *holidays* if you are going to speak about these.

Suggestions — to the deafened: Learn to *concentrate* your hearing;

Try to find a trained therapist to give you auditory training so that you learn to recognize the new sounds you hear;

Try to have practice in picking out one sound from a background noise.

If speech is clear and the lipreader is attentive, then the

clues obtained from eye and ear will be relayed to the mind. But sense will only be made if the following conditions apply:

The speaker — has good mouth movements,
            — has spoken in a clear tone of voice,
            — has given a clue or sufficient context for the mind to make an intelligent appraisal.

The listener — has been able to read some lipreading shapes,
            — has been able to gauge the rhythm of the sentence,
            — has been able to relay clues to the mind and use experience and knowledge of his language to reply sensibly.

All this appears to happen very quickly with good lipreaders.

However, we must remember how long it takes to become a good ballet dancer or violinist, how much practice is needed daily, how many rungs there are on the ladder to perfection, how much less one would expect if either skill was taken up at the age of sixty-plus, and the peculiarity of lipreading. This last point is that the lipreader cannot use his skill until he is fed information — the violinist can find pleasure in playing to himself, the dancer can dance round the room with joy, but the lipreader is dependent on *you* and *the way you speak*. The cleverest lipreader in the world cannot understand an immobile face that is managing to speak through its teeth at 140 words a minute.

Suggestions for Practice

I doubt that you can practise on your own. Yes, you can watch your face in a mirror to see what your own mouth does when you make certain shapes, but this defeats the main purpose of lipreading — to be able to make some sense from a stranger's face without any mental clue as to what he may say.

Also, I do believe that we all need another person, or the stimulus of a group, to keep going. The beginnings of any skill are sheer donkey work and it is all too easy to give up when you are on your own.

Try to find a helper
Despite the fact that it is your wife and family that you will probably lipread most, they are not always the best helpers. A wife who has worked all day with you in mind, doing her housework, shopping and cooking, is not coming to a practice session in the best of moods if she has just had to wash up, and would rather put her feet up and read or watch television. There are exceptions and, if couples are retired, then they are likely to have time during mornings or afternoons when they can sit together and use material. But most lipreaders have either to find a class or club with practice sessions, or a friend who will be more detached and, therefore, more able to criticize kindly and encourage.

Sit across a table from your helper or face each other in chairs about four to six feet apart, with light on the speaker's face. When you have had several sessions together then try moving the chairs a little further apart, or angle them to see the speaker in part-profile, as it often helps to see a jaw movement from the side. It is not an eating session so leave all refreshment until you feel you both deserve it afterwards; you won't have to wait long because no session should be longer than half an hour to start with, and it is better to have two or three shorter sessions each week than one long, tiring practice.

Watching people practise together, it usually happens that they get to a sticking point where all the helper can do is to keep repeating the same thing, either because there is no alternative phrase to use, or she can think of none. For this reason it is better to have a table between you and some paper, so that the friend can write down the troublesome word. Not being a teacher, she is unlikely to know which sound or phrase is the problem but with practice she will begin to realize that the same difficulties occur time and time again. Keep these papers for further practice — it is the difficulties that need revision.

The helper
Do not worry that you feel awkward at the start. You *will* feel worried if your deaf friend is unable to lipread you well; you may feel irritated that he doesn't seem to read obvious things; and you may feel embarrassed that he appears to stare at your mouth so much. It will not be easy

reading material that has been devised by someone else and which sometimes appears unnecessary or futile. But all these feelings pass. If you speak clearly and carefully, but as naturally as possible, and avoid speaking too quickly, you will put the material across very well. Read it through first yourself so that you have an idea of phrasing — you don't want to umm and er in the middle of a sentence — and keep to your natural rhythm of speech so that the sentences come out smoothly.

Don't try to 'devoice'. If your friend is severely deaf then he won't hear your voice at the distance; if he wears an aid then the background of your voice helps to give the rhythm and stress of your sentences, and it has been shown that devoicing always produces some degree of distortion of the mouth. Be prepared to repeat and repeat. If your friend has read something easily, repeat it to give him pleasure and confidence. If he has read a piece badly, repeat it for practice, although not necessarily at the same session; keep it until the next time and have a further try. You will soon be teaching yourself — realizing what difficulties to expect when you pre-read the material and becoming more adept at changing phrases into more lipreadable language. When this stage has been reached, then try not to write anything down. Make yourself think of another way round a phrase and see if your friend can get this before returning to the original that meant much the same.

Try not to move your arms about, keep the script away from your face, and try not to read looking down at the paper but hold a sentence in your mind, look up and say it. Have a pre-arranged code where you just nod if the lipreader is correct and shake your head otherwise, but don't go into long explanations or chat as this diverts attention from the material and is confusing.

It would require an entire book to give lessons around all the visible shapes. The following exercises are meant to set a lipreader on the road to his skill which, if practised regularly, will produce a watching and thinking attitude.

I will include some more difficult material, which can be used equally well with beginners if more clues are given throughout the exercises.

Explanations are kept brief since all we are expecting is that the helper will have no theoretical knowledge and will merely be reading a script. A copy of the script should be looked at by the reader first — he is never going to memorize it and it saves the need for writing down an explanation of what is coming. And if he sees 'Numbers' then he is immediately tuned in.

Numbers

So let us start with number work — always necessary when asking times, or bus routes, or for money and shopping purposes.

Number shapes

one	(look for wun)
two	(also to, too)
three	(visible th)
four	(also for, fore)
five	(f/v alike)
six	(little movement)
seven	(look for 2 syllables, good v)
eight	(also ate, jaw drops)
nine	(difficult to distinguish from each other)
and ten	
eleven	(visible l and v)
twelve	(visible w and v)

The reader should mix these up after showing each shape twice and then ask lipreader to give back each number.

Now pick it out of a sentence: She bought four loaves. (Then six/three/eight/two.)

We asked twelve friends to the party. (Then five/seven/twelve/eleven.)

Add time — half-past, quarter-to, quarter-past, o'clock.
We asked them to come at half-past five.
We asked them to come at half-past seven.
We asked them to come at eight o'clock.
We asked them to come at six.
They left at about eleven.
They left at about a quarter to one.
They left at about half-past twelve.
They left at about a quarter to two.

The lipreader should *always* repeat what he reads — *never* accept a nod for an answer since in lipreading so much can be misread out of context.

You cannot say that you have learned numbers until you can recognize them within a context. In the following piece, look at it first, then try to 'see' the numbers as they come along, without trying to get all the other words exactly.

One dark winter evening *two* people stopped at a village. They had walked more than *three miles* through pouring rain. They had started their walk over *four* hours ago. They'd had nothing to eat *for five* hours. They saw a pub in the village called The *Six* Bells so they went inside. The landlord said that supper would be ready by *seven* o'clock. There were *eight* people at supper and it was well after *nine* before the meal was finished. They were given room number *ten* and were so worn out that they were both in bed well before *eleven*.

It is possible to repeat this piece changing the numbers round if the speaker alters his script.

There is little use in learning numbers and not being able to lipread the word number itself. So look at:

I number him among my best friends.

There are a number of things I must do this morning.

I've told him not to do that, time without number.

I could feel my shoulder growing number after that blow he gave me. (Number — different sound, same shape.)

Then add an ordinal number onto some common phrase if you aren't running out of concentration:

That's the third/fourth/second time I've told him.

We have our meetings on the first/second/third/fourth Tuesday of each month.

He didn't do badly — he came sixth/tenth/seventh/eighth in his class.

There are a number of things I must do this morning. First, I must leave a note for the milkman because I want two extra pints. Then I want to get to the butcher when he opens at half-past eight and buy four or five chops for this evening. I know you'll say that's the second time we've had chops this week but I shan't be home until after six and they won't take more than seven minutes to fry.

What about collective numbers?

There are a number of things I have to do this morning.

I have a score of letters to type.

There are half a dozen people that I must ring.

There are a hundred pamphlets to deliver for the church bazaar and I have a million jobs to do about the house.

Drill: score/hundred/dozen/million.

Repeat each word twice, pause and repeat the next. Then carefully mix them, using each two or three times and when you stop ask which was the last one you said. This will allow the eye to take in the few clues in all these words.

Important points on number

The teens and tens are similar in shape to the lipreader, that is, thirteen will resemble thirty, fourteen resemble forty and so on. With useful residual hearing it is likely that the wearer of an aid will hear the nasal ending of the teens, fifteen, sixteen, and the rest but, if unsure, it is always better to ask the speaker, 'Did you say thirty?' rather than 'What did you say?'. In this way you will receive a clear Yes/No answer and be certain of which is meant.

Numbers need listening practice also. It is easy to differentiate three and four on the lips but less easy when trying to hear on the telephone. Similarly with thirty and forty — this is because the vowel sounds are liable to distortion and may sound very alike.

Useful Drills

Here are a few useful drills which can be done at any time for a short practice or to gain a little speed in lipreading. They give repetition on a phrase which has its own rhythm or the final words may be used alone to show different shape changes.

It put me off my food/my stroke/my work/balance.

Didn't he look well!/washed out/brown/ill.

Can you manage next weekend?/Wednesday/month/week.

The only difference between week/weekend will be a jaw

movement and beginners should start looking for such clues as soon as possible.

I'll go to the market tomorrow/on Tuesday/today.

Try this the other way round
Tomorrow I'll go to the market
On Tuesday I'll go to the market
Today I'll go to the market.
Are you going out this morning/afternoon/evening?
Are you going out later?

Now lengthen each sentence:
Are you going out this morning — if so bring me back some stamps.
Are you going out this afternoon — if so please take my book back to the library for me.
Are you going out this evening — if so, I'll get you to post a letter for me.
Are you going out later — if so, I'd like to come with you.
I can't manage Thursday/Saturday/Monday/Friday.

Now lengthen:
I can't manage Friday, I'm already booked up.
I can't manage Saturday, it's a busy day for me.
I can't manage Monday, it's too short notice.
I can't manage Thursday, I have to visit someone in hospital.

Now put the day first:
Friday will be alright for me, I can leave work early.
Saturday will be alright for me, I shall be free then.
Monday will be alright for me, I can leave the dog with my neighbour.
Thursday will be alright for me, I've nothing else to do.

Problems with days
All weekdays, excepting Saturday, have good initial shapes, but Saturday and Sunday can be distinguished only by rhythm or slight extra jaw movement and when unsure the lipreader should ask, 'Did you say Sunday?' and get a Yes/No answer.

Saturday resembles 'yesterday' but frequently Saturday is preceded by 'On', a word we never attach to yesterday.

Watching Practice

This section is no more than watching practice. Each line is based on using the same root letters and changing either the initial, medial or final consonant or vowel. Even without a teacher present, a lipreader will see the change in shape from one word to the next as his helper repeats them, slowly at first and then with more speed. No more than two lines should be practised at any one time and they are useful 'warming up' exercises as well as encouraging full concentration.

Initial consonant change

fish	wish	dish	
fall	shawl	pall	
thank	tank	lank	

(note that only the initial consonant is visible)

father	rather	lather	
thin	gin	pin	

(note that only the *first* consonant is visible)

bill	will	fill	rill
peer	leer	veer	

Medial consonant and vowel change

reheat	repeat	reseat
produce	profuse	
barn	boon	bean
board	bird	bead
potter	patter	putter
reshape	reship	
father	farmer	
tip	tap	top

Final change

rope	role	rove	
leaf	leash	leap	
both	boat	bole	
batch	bash	badge	
mad	lad	fad	sad

The helper could tick any combination that appears especially difficult, to repeat at each session. She should also encourage the lipreader to *say* the words himself, after he has read them, to encourage a kinaesthetic tie-up with the visual.

Conversation Retention

We need to encourage retention of conversation in case the lipreader is asked a question at the end. At the start of a skill it is common to be so attentive on the analytic that the whole meaning is not stored away. A few minutes practice on the following encourages concentration and retention of what is being said. Try one in each session.

Retention and recall:
I've got a rather grubby hanky in my pocket.
I've got a rather grubby hanky and some loose change.
I've got a rather grubby hanky, some loose change and a sweet wrapper.
What do I have?

When I'm out I must make a telephone call.
When I'm out I must make a telephone call and go to the bank.
When I'm out I must make a telephone call, go to the bank and then do some shopping.
What have I got to do?

Poor Barbara cut her lip when she fell on the pavement.
Poor Barbara cut her lip when she fell on the pavement and bruised one side of her face.
Poor Barbara cut her lip when she fell on the pavement, bruised the side of her face and broke her spectacles.
What did she do to herself?

Bob has just retired from work.
Bob has just retired from work and potters around the house.
Bob has just retired from work and potters around the house or does a bit in the garden.
Bob has just retired from work and potters around the house or just does a bit in the garden and drives his wife mad.
What does he do?

An Interesting Story

Stories are always appreciated by lipreaders because in many ways they are easier than the single sentence — so long as the reader can stay with the speaker, enough clues can be gathered to get at least the gist of the tale. However, a story unattached to a teaching point seems a waste of opportunity and it is possible to use the tale, or a joke, a topic, or a rhyme, as basis for teaching points. The following is one example of this. Remember to let the lipreader see the script first since there is no teacher present to pick up points as he goes along.

A man found his false teeth uncomfortable so he took them out and put them on the table. When he went back for them a few hours later he couldn't find them. He walked round the house looking for his teeth, although he was sure that he had left them on the table in the kitchen. He opened the back door and saw his large Labrador dog sitting on the patio. When the dog turned round it had the teeth firmly fixed in its mouth. The dog must have pulled them off the table and now it was grinning like a Cheshire Cat. The man tried to pull them from the dog's mouth but couldn't so he had to take the animal to the vet. The teeth had to be removed under an anaesthetic. Would you believe it!

Teaching points
How do we use the word *believe* in everyday language?
  Try to lipread these expressions:
  Would you believe it!
  Would *you* believe it!
  I don't believe a word of it.
  I can't believe it!
  It's beyond belief.

Now look again as the speaker says them and watch for facial clues.

Repetition
It's easy to believe that where there's a will there's a way.
It's easy to believe that every cloud has a silver lining.
It's easy to believe that it never rains but what it pours.
It's easy to believe that all's well that ends well.

It's difficult to believe that if you laugh, the world laughs with you.
It's difficult to believe that a rolling stone gathers no moss.
It's difficult to believe that a bird in the hand is worth two in the bush.
It's difficult to believe a little learning is a dangerous thing.

This may provoke some discussion.

How belief is used:
Mrs Bradford told me/that to the *best of her belief*/the new
vicar has thirteen children/but I really can't believe that.

The council announced that/contrary to public belief/the
rates would be going up/to a figure *beyond the realms of
belief*.

I believe you said you would help/at the church fair next
Saturday/but we have so many volunteers/that *it's my belief*
it won't be necessary thank you.

Other words indicating belief:
Drill: Are you sure? Are you certain? Are you positive?
Yes, I'm sure/certain/positive.
No, I'm not sure/certain/positive, but I think so.

Many things we believe in are old wives' tales. In the book
Alice in Wonderland, the Queen said that it is *easy to
believe* in impossible things but it is important *to be aware*
that they *are* impossible. Alice said, 'There's no use trying.
One *can't believe* impossible things.' The Queen replied, 'I
daresay you haven't had enough practice. When I was your
age I always did it for half an hour a day. Why, sometimes *I
believed* as many as six impossible things before breakfast.'

Can you see a difference: look at, beware, be aware.

Mental tie-up
When you cross a field beware of the bull.
When you enter a farm gate beware of the dog.
When you swim in the River Nile beware of the crocodiles.
When you come to a level crossing beware of the trains.
Before you take out insurance be aware of the conditions.
Before you climb a mountain be aware of the dangers.
Before you have to break some bad news be aware of other
people's feelings.
Before you plan a holiday abroad be aware of the rate of
exchange.

Stories for the More Practised Lipreader
For the more practised reader — choose one piece to do in
a session.

Sometimes our cherished beliefs/are shattered:
Cinderella wore glass slippers — all children believe this
but in the first version of the story Cinderella wore slippers

of fur. The story was French and the French word for fur is vair. When the story was rewritten in the fourteenth century the writer mistook vair (spell this out) for verre (spell out) which means glass. So Cinderella was given a glass slipper. Would you believe it!

We believe that snakes are charmed by music — this cannot be true because snakes have no ears. They cannot hear sounds which are airborne. They may be influenced by the vibrations of the charmer's foot tapping on the ground. When they are out of the basket they will respond to the swaying of the body and the pipe. Would you believe it!

We believe that lightning never strikes twice in the same place. This is quite untrue. Lightning generally strikes prominent buildings or tall trees. As long as they remain prominent then lightning will tend to strike them. The Empire State Building was struck sixty-eight times during its first ten years and a lot of English churches have been struck several times. Because of this high buildings have a lightning conductor, which is a copper rod. This is a good conductor of electricity. If it is hit it will carry the electrical charge down to earth. Would you believe it!

And another unbelievable story:

A woman boarded a bus in America with nine children. When the conductor came she gave him her fare and one penny for one of the children. She then produced the family Bible to show that all but one of her children were under five years of age. She had triplets of four years nine months; twins aged three and a half; another set of twins aged two years and a baby of nine months. She showed the conductor that all their names began with the letter A. The eldest was Alice; the triplets were April, Amy, and Angela; the twin boys were Arthur and Adrian and the other pair were Alan and Amon; and the baby was called Agatha. Would you believe it!

Let us return to some simple phrases and see whether the expression used by the speaker gives any clues:

I can't believe — she's almost eighty.
　　　　　　　　— the summer is almost over.
　　　　　　　　— it's taken me two hours to get here.

How does it look the other way round?
  She's almost eighty — I can't believe it!
  The summer is almost over — I can't believe it!
  It's taken me two hours to get here — I can't believe it!

Another word connected with belief is 'true', which will look like rue on the lips.

Practise: Is it true that you're moving shortly?
  Is it true that you're leaving us?
  Is it true that your wife is in hospital?

Try these another way round:
  I heard that you're moving shortly — is it true?
  I heard that you're leaving us — is it true?
  I heard that your wife is in hospital — is it true?

More eye drill: I can't believe that/credit that/understand that/accept that.

Now try the following, having first looked at your script, then try to get these unrelated stories first time.

Would you believe it?
Henry the First decided that the measure for one yard should be the distance from his nose to his outstretched thumb. (Difficulties will be decided, yard, distance, and nose.)

A woman woke up to find the dead body of a man wedged in her bedroom window. The police found out that he was a burglar who had died from a heart attack. (Difficulties will be dead, man, had died, and attack.)

President Truman was once very bored at a reception where he had to shake hands with hundreds of people. So every time he shook hands he muttered, 'I murdered my grandmother this morning.' Nobody blinked on eyelash, except one man who growled back, 'She had it coming to her.' (Difficulties are was, once, shake hands, hundreds, muttered, murdered, an eyelash, except, back, and had it coming.)

The opposite of true is *false* and this will look like *force* to a lipreader. Context is often helpful to sort out a meaning.
  There is no force behind his statement.

He made a false statement.
He played without any force behind his strokes.
He played her false.

Many of us wear something false. There is a story about a
man who married his girlfriend and watched her undress on
their wedding night. First she took off her false eyelashes,
then she removed her contact lenses, then her auburn wig,
then her false teeth, and then her falsies. He ran out of the
room, horrified, crying, 'You false wretch, you are not the
woman I married!' Would you believe it!

Finally, here are remarks which may be said to you — try to
get them first time.
    You can't believe a word they say!
    It's just not true.
    He/she is not telling the truth.
    That's the truth of it.
    I never heard a truer word spoken.
    We can't always recognize the truth when we hear it.
    That is a downright lie.
    He lies through his teeth. (Lie has little shape but the
    context will probably allow you to guess it.)

The Sound of Words
We should do a lesson to show that spelling should be
ignored and thought given to the sound of words.
    Look at — *cough, bough, dough, through, tough,* and you
will see that the first and last end in the shape of f and the
other words not only have no f ending but also present
vowel changes.

Let's look at cough:
Remember it wasn't the cough that carried him off.
It was the coffin they carried him off in.

Repetition:
There are cough mixtures to take in the morning.
There are cough mixtures to take at night.
There are cough mixtures to take after every meal.
There are cough mixtures to suppress the cough.
There are cough mixtures to soothe a tickle.
There are cough mixtures to relieve congestion.
There are cough mixtures flavoured with menthol.

There are cough mixtures flavoured with lemon and honey.
There are cough mixtures strong enough to give to a horse.
There are cough mixtures weak enough to give to babies.

Longer piece:
But according to the specialists at the London Chest
Hospital, all cough mixtures are useless — they do not cure
a cough. They say if you have a cough and take some
medicine it will take one week to lose the cough. If you
have a cough and don't take medicine it will take seven
days for the cough to go! So, what do these specialists
recommend? They rely on the good old-fashioned methods
of steam inhalation. They say boil some water and simply
breathe in the steam. You can drop in a few drops of
menthol if you want. Boots the Chemists agree with these
remarks but they say people would not believe it if they
were told there was nothing for their cough.
    What do you take if you have a cough?

Colloquial use:
My brother wanted to go on holiday with us but I told him
he would have to *cough up the money* first.
He just stood there, twisting his hands and saying nothing,
so I finally got impatient with him and said *"Cough it up."*
We have just had to *cough out* for more repairs to the car.

Drill: He's had a terrible cough/hacking cough/rasping
cough/tickling cough.

In listening practice you will have difficulties with the
proximity of vowels in cough/cuff/calf. But it is often the
adjective before the word that will give a clue.
    He has a bad cough/dirty cuff/newborn calf. (Not likely to
be newborn cough or cuff.)

Involvement using cough/bough/dough/through (but drill
these first).
Tell me something that makes you cough.
Tell me which end of the ship is the bow.
Tell me what you would do if you came into a lot of dough.
Tell me something you would put through the eye of a
needle. (Or a letterbox, for beginners.)
Tell me a tree that has its boughs close to the ground.
Tell me for which charity would you cough up some
money.

Tell me anything that can be made from dough when your wife is working with it in the kitchen.

Tell me what runs through your head when you're asked these questions?

Practical

It is usually possible in a home to collect a few things from about the house to put on a tray — things revolving round the lesson.

For example, if you found a tin of cough sweets or a bottle of cough mixture, a postcard, a rolling pin, a hair bow, you could ask the lipreader to point to the object in answer to:

What would I use if I had a bad cough?

What would I use to roll out some dough?

Which would I put through a letterbox?

Which would I wear in my hair?

Mental tie-up

This is to encourage the lipreader to continue to the end of the sentence so that if the start is missed he may well find the clue in the last part.

I use a sweet dough to make a fruit flan.

I use a sour dough to make sour bread.

I use plain dough to make a pie crust.

I use an unleavened dough to make flat bread.

I use a rich dough to make flaky pastry.

I use watery dough to make a cold water paste.

If this is not especially relevant to a man then try the following:

I put a note through her letterbox because she didn't answer the bell.

I put some string round the catch to stop the window from banging.

I put a pipe cleaner through my ear mould to remove the wax.

I put a comb through my hair to make it tidy.

I put a piece of strong thread through the needle to mend my leather slippers.

I put my foot through the door to stop her banging it in my face.

I put a mark through the question to show that I'd answered it.

Colours

Colour is important in everyday language as will be seen from the following examples. It is good and simple practice to drill the common colours, although finally it is the word 'colour' itself which presents the greatest problem to the lipreader — watch yourself say, 'I like the colour' and you will realize how little shape there is.

This lesson is meant to cover practice both in this word and in everyday use of colour.

We have warm colours — red, orange, yellow, pink, brown.

Let the reader see these twice and then mix them up and let him repeat what you have said.

We have cold colours — blue, green, grey.

Green and grey look very similar on some mouths and may also be confused with red because the initial letter g is not visible on the lips.

When colours are mixed with *white* we have tints such as cream, pale blue, and pale green. When colours are mixed with *black* we have tones such as dark red, navy blue, and brown.

On bright sunny days all colours look stronger and brighter than they do on a dull day. So we associate some colours with feelings:

She looks blue with cold.

She's green with envy.

She's purple with anger.

Can you pick out the colour now from the following?
Yesterday was a *red*-letter day for Mrs Roberts. She woke up feeling *blue*. It was a wet, *grey* morning — enough to put anyone in a *black* mood. But Mrs Roberts had to go to work, however *browned* off she felt. She waited more than twenty minutes for a bus and reached the office *purple* with cold. Her fingers were *white* to the tips. Her secretary brought her a steaming cup of *black* coffee which brought the *pink* back into her cheeks. Then she opened her post. The first letter was in a *buff* envelope and she went as *white* as a sheet when she saw what was inside — she had won a Premium Bond prize. She saw the world through *rose-*

coloured spectacles once more. The girls in the office were *green* with envy but said they would go out with her that evening and paint the town *red*.

Some people suffer from colour blindness.
There are more men who are colour blind than there are women.
The most common form of colour blindness is when a person can see no difference between red and green (rather like the lipreading problem).
To these people both red and green may look blue, or grey, or a yellowish colour.

Think of some of the problems they might have, such as trying to work out traffic lights.

If you are colour blind you cannot join the Navy.
If you are colour blind you cannot drive a bus or a train.
If you are colour blind you cannot work in a paint factory.
If you are colour blind you cannot play Ludo.
If you are colour blind you cannot work in a florist's.

If you have an eye for colour you could be an interior decorator.
If you have an eye for colour you could be an artist.
If you have an eye for colour you could be a dress designer.
If you have an eye for colour you could be a milliner.
If you have an eye for colour you could be a landscape gardener.

Do you have an eye for colour?
If you wore a dark blue suit and a white shirt — what colour tie would you wear?
If your house was red brick with a grey roof — what colour would you paint your front door?
If your wife wanted orange curtains and a brown carpet — what colour would you paint the walls?
If you had red roses and yellow marigolds in one bed — what colour flowers would you grow on the wall behind?

Colloquial use:
I like red — it's such a cheerful colour.
I like brown — you can wear so many other colours with it.

I like yellow — it makes me feel bright and sunny.
I don't care for black — it makes me look an old hag.
I don't care for pink — it reminds me of cream fondants.
I don't care for orange — it's too startling for my taste.

My brother said he would buy my old black car. I said to him. 'First, show me the *colour of your money.*'

I went out last night to a Chinese restaurant and had a huge meal. That's probably why I feel *off colour* this morning.

We took my aunt to the seaside after her operation. After a few days the fresh air brought the *colour back* into her cheeks.

Drill on difficult combinations: That's a peculiar/hectic/startling/an unusual/a garish colour.
Repeat and mix.

Can you recognize the song title and pick out the colour?
We all live in a yellow submarine.
I'm dreaming of a white Christmas.
John Brown's body lies a-mouldering in the grave.
There'll be blue birds over the white cliffs of Dover.
Ten green bottles hanging on the wall.
There's a rainbow round my shoulder and the sky is blue above.
Tie a yellow ribbon round the old oak tree.
I'm sending red roses to a blue lady.
Darling, I am growing old, silver threads among the gold.

Let us look at 'gold', which is similar to other words on the lips. Watch yourself say old, hold, cold, sold, and even told, and you will find them alike. You can but trust that context will sort them out for you but it is not always so. 'He's given me a gold watch' might well be, 'He's given me an old watch'. But in, 'I bought an old-gold bedspread' there is no difficulty.

You may be wearing a gold watch, a gold ring, a gold necklace or chain, a pair of gold earrings, all of which could be old. But you will have a cold in the head (not gold) and no hold on your emotions and an old pair of shoes that are comfortable.

Longer piece
An elderly couple were celebrating their golden wedding.

The family were arranging a party for them and bringing presents made of gold. The two grandchildren also wanted to buy something to give to their grandparents but when they went to the shops they found all the gold articles cost more than they could afford. Then the boy had a bright idea. He took his sister to the local market. When they arrived at the party they gave their grandparents a large bag. Grandmother opened it and she brought out one pound of Golden Delicious apples, two packets of Golden Wonder crisps, one tin of Golden Syrup, one packet of golden fish fingers, a pack of golden bread crumbs, and a jar of Golden Shred marmalade.

Grannie was so touched that she wept golden tears.

The following Colour Quiz is to encourage a quick answer from the lipreader. In the early stages he is likely to repeat back what is said to him. A more advanced stage is when he is able to absorb the question, think of the answer and come out with this immediately. This is one way of judging the ability of a lipreader as it is difficult to devise a practical test.

A quiz is not easy, since there is little connected theme to relate to but it is usually enjoyed and encourages a quick response.

What colour is a roll of kitchen foil?
What colour is an ounce of tobacco?
What colour is raw meat?
What colour is a boiled lobster?
What colour is a bunch of ripe bananas?
What colour is the fibre of a coconut?
What colour is the lining of a cloud?
What colour is a pine cone?

This second quiz brings in six unreadable words which may be guessed from the final word in each sentence. Such exercises show that adults are able to use their store of language to make intelligent guesses — in fact they often feel they have lipread the unlipreadable word!

What colour is the *centre* of a walnut?
What colour is the *hide* of an elephant?
What colour is the *stone* of a peach?
What colour is the *tongue* of a Chow?

What colour is the *inside* of an avocado pear?
What colour is the *skin* of a Granny Smith apple?

Return to colour and the emotions
Blue is said to be a cold colour — so don't paint your bathroom blue.
Red is said to be a hot colour — so don't paint the summerhouse red.
White is said to be a pure colour — so brides wear white on their wedding day.
Black is said to be a mysterious colour — so women outline their eyes with black.

   Now let us concentrate on one colour — brown.   This is a more difficult piece but may still be tackled by the less advanced if they have read the copy first.

   Remember they should repeat each phrase so that the helper can check mistakes.

Sir Samuel Browne was born in India in 1824. He was the son of a British army surgeon. He spent most of his career in Britain and India, in the army. He was awarded the Victoria Cross for his courage in capturing an enemy gun and stopping it from firing upon the advancing infantry. During the hand-to-hand fighting he received two wounds, one in the left leg and the other in his left shoulder. He recovered but had trouble in wearing his sword. The sword hung on the left side of his belt for full dress wear and Browne needed a left arm to hold it up when he walked. To solve the problem he made himself a special belt for everyday use. This was balanced by a strap running across his chest from the opposite shoulder. Other army officers started to copy this and in 1900 the belt was actually included in regulations for service dress.

So many things are brown:
   A horse chestnut fruit is brown.
   A plot of earth is brown.
   The hide of a Jersey cow is brown.
   The bark of an oak tree is brown.
   The mud at the bottom of a stream is brown.
   A piece of seaweed is brown.
   The shell of a coconut is brown.
   The leaves of a copper beech are brown.

A lobster shell is brown.

I feel browned off after all that.

Requiring a quick answer:
Tell me a fruit that is yellow.
Tell me a bird that is blue.
Tell me a vegetable that is purple.
Tell me a flower that is orange.
Tell me an animal that is brown.
Tell me a food that is white.
Tell me a fish that is red.
Tell me an insect that is green.
Tell me a butterfly that is white.
Tell me a sweet that is black and white.

Now to return to our problem of old/gold/cold/sold and told.
Tell me something that feels cold.
Tell me something made of gold.
Tell me something you were told as a child.
Tell me something you can hold on to.
Tell me something that may be sold in a greengrocers.
Tell me something that you won't be able to do when you're old.
Tell me something that you would *behold* as you approached New York.

Small articles of the same colour can be put on a tray and the helper say, 'Show me the blue pen/the blue book/the blue toothbrush/the blue tissue/the blue cotton/the blue dishcloth.' The helper can give further simple practice on all colours in this way.

Short Exercises
Five minute repetitive exercises if you haven't any more time to spare.

Repeat the phrase in *italics* each time.

What did he do? He came home late.
He stayed out all night.
He quarrelled with his boss.
He lost his job.
He smashed up his car.

He resigned from the team.
He spent all his money.
He spent all her money.

What did she do? She bought a new hat.
She had a coffee morning.
She took the children to school.
She arranged the flowers in church.
She went to the hairdressers.
She joined a dressmaking class.
She went to Aerobics.

It must be ten years since I saw you. What have you been doing?

Since I saw you I've got married.
found another job.
sold my house.
moved away.
joined the Police.
written a book.
brought up a family.
been abroad.

For a mental tie-up
My head feels so heavy I can't think properly.
My eyes are so tired I can't read properly.
My nose is so stuffy I can't breathe properly.
My leg is so stiff I can't walk properly.
My throat is so sore I can't talk properly.
My back is so painful I can't stand properly.
My chest is so thick I can't sleep properly.

I can't think properly because I have no concentration.
I can't breathe properly because I have asthma.
I can't talk properly because I have a lisp.
I can't sleep properly because I have bad dreams.
I can't walk properly because I have a bunion.
I can't read properly because the light is so bad.

Probably and properly look alike. Try to sort them out in these sentences.
I'm properly fed up about it.
It will probably snow tomorrow.
He performed his duties most properly.

He has been properly brought up.
I am probably quite mistaken.
I wish you would lay the table properly.

Presenting Material

There are as many ways to present material on lipreading as
there are teachers with ideas. One of the more usual ways to
present lipreading shapes in class is through isolating each
shape, with its similarities. For instance a session would be
taken to show that p/b/m make similar lipreading shapes.

I have found, since learning is done a little at a time, that
it is helpful to present one of these letters at a time and then
do a final session using all three, so that the lipreader has
spent four sessions on the same theme. An example of this
would be a general introduction to the sounds, showing
some peculiarities, followed by one lesson mainly on one of
the sounds — in this case m, although naturally it is never
possible to eliminate the other two p/b entirely.

With a helper, both should read the introductory remarks
on the sounds before using the practice material.

P, B, M. The letters we call Pea, Bee, and Em, are sounded
in speech as Pa as in paper, Ba as in baby, and Ma as in
marmalade. If you look as you say these three sounds you
will notice that the lips come together and then explode the
air outwards. The shapes are similar, although the sounds
are different: pa is a voiceless explosion of air; ba can be
heard as it is voiced; and ma has a nasal quality.

However, to the lipreader words such as pill, bill, and
mill, will look alike. This applies also to words starting with
ap, ab, and am — apple/amble/approach/a brooch, and to
doublings such as pl, bl, pr, br — planned/bland/
pride/bride.

When two of these shapes come together, only one
movement is made. For example, I must com*b my* hair/my
jo*b m*ust come first.

Before a p,b, or m, assimilation may take place as the mouth
is economizing on movements.

For example, bag and baggage — bag am baggage, that is,
another sound is changed to a p, b or m shape. Football may
sound like foopball. These assimiliations may not take
place; it varies according to the speed of speech and who is
talking.

Watch yourself say these over and over and you will feel
what is meant and see what happens:
come back, come back — ends up sounding the same as
comeback.
warm milk, warm milk — almost becomes warmilk.

It might help to know, if you have to make a guess, that m
appears more often at the start of words then either p or b.
So let us start with m and see how it appears in different
positions.

It is clearly visible at the start of a word — more more
more. Also in the medial position — lumber, lumber (even
though it is with b it makes only the single shape), and it is
clearly visible at the end — name name name.
Unfortunately the last could easily be read as *aim* and it
would be difficult to distinguish between 'I didn't
understand his name, did you?' and 'I didn't understand his
aim, did you?'

Let us do some repetition using 'more'. Mix the following
and ask the reader to repeat:

We would all like more money
We would all like more time to spare
We would all like more leisure time
We would all like more peace of mind

Longer piece for imagination to come into play. Keep
looking for the m's.

Mrs Morris was a happy woman. She was in good health.
She had a kind husband. She had three lovely children. She
had a beautiful home. Sometimes she said to herself 'What
more could I want?'

Mrs Miller was a very unhappy woman. Every week she
seemed to have more problems. Every week there seemed
more washing to do, more bills to pay, mouths to feed and
less time to do them. Sometimes she said to herself, 'Surely,
nothing more can happen!'

Well, we don't want any more of that, we've had more
than enough.

Let us see m in the middle of lumber — although not truly
in the middle for the lipreader since 'er' becomes a neutral a
in sound.

Most houses have a lumber room. We lumber ourselves with all sorts of old junk. Recently I turned out my lumber room.

Amongst the lumber I found my mother's shawl.
Amongst the lumber I found a pile of empty match boxes.
Amongst the lumber I found a mound of old postcards.
Amongst the lumber I found a broken musical box.
Amongst the lumber I found a mildewed chest.
Amongst the lumber I found a box of mothballs.

Most of the lumber I shall give to the next jumble sale.

If you have a lot of lumber at home then you can give it to Oxfam or burn it or leave it out for the dustmen. However, if you have a pain in your lumbar region then it is wise to go and see your doctor.

Name
Here are some phrases you may need to lipread.
What did you say your name was?
I didn't quite catch your name.
I still haven't caught your name.
Would you mind repeating your name.
What's her name?
What's his name?
That's old what's-his-name.
He wouldn't leave his name.

Drill: He has a very peculiar name.
       He has a very unusual name.
       He has a very common name.
       He has a very appropriate name.

A man named Thomas Fuller wrote in the seventeenth century that a name is a kind of face. Names are very interesting. In the past we had only one name each.

Some people were named after the places where they lived — we all know a Mr Hill, a Mr Ford, and a Mr Upton (uptown).

Some people were named after animals — we all know a Mr Fox, a Mr Hart, and a Mr Wolf.

Some people were named after colours — we all know a Mr White, a Mr Brown, and a Mr Black.

Some people were named after their characteristics — we all know a Mr Bright, a Mr Merry, and a Mr Smart.

Some people were named after their trade or craft — we all know a Mr Smith, a Mr Baker, and a Mr Fletcher (maker of arrows).

People have been named after rivers, mountains, flowers, trees, jewels, wars, or the circumstances of their birth. For example, Moses received his name because he had been left in an ark among the bulrushes. When the daughter of Pharaoh found him she called him Moses, because she drew him out of the water — mo is water and ushr means saved.

People give their houses some very strange names:

Every day a man passed a house named Maldeb. (*Write this down*). He often wondered what it meant. One morning he saw a woman coming out so he plucked up courage to ask. 'Oh', she said, 'We have seven children, two dogs, two cats and a hamster, so our house is Bedlam back to front.'

One couple said that a few years ago they were thrilled to be able to buy their own house after living in rooms for many years. They proudly named it 'Charnel', from the husband's name Charles and the wife's name Nelly. However, they changed it quickly when a neighbour told them to look in the dictionary and they found that a charnel house contained bones.

One house that is opposite the local maternity hospital has a most appropriate name. It is called 'Swell View'.

And a newly married couple named their house 'Grafton Grind' because they said that is what they had to do to get it — hard work and doing without.

The word 'nickname' is interesting. In Old English the word was eke-name, meaning other name. The extra piece put on the bottom of a beehive is still called an eke. Try some names — if you lipread the nationality then you will be able to guess the nickname.

The nickname for an Irishman is Paddy.

The nickname for a Scot is Mac or Sandy.

The nickname for a Welshman is Taffy.

The nickname for a Frenchman is Froggie.

The nickname for a German is Fritz or Jerry.

The nickname for a Portuguese is Dago.

The nickname for an English soldier is Tommy Atkins. This is because soldiers had to fill in an identity book during the First World War. To show them how to do this a sample form was produced and the name chosen for the form was Tommy Atkins.

Contracted names are more difficult to lipread because they are shorter than the full name. Try the following and wait until you see the full name appear, when you will probably guess what went before. You will often be doing this in lipreading.

The full name for Tom is Thomas.
The full name for Ted is Edward.
The full name for Jeff is Geoffrey.
The full name for Dick is Richard.
The full name for Les is Leslie.
The full name for Bill is William.
The full name for Bob is Robert.
The full name for Hal is Henry.
The full name for Pat is Patricia.
The full name for Penny is Penelope.
The full name for Bea is Beatrice.
The full name for Kate is Katherine.
The full name for Phyl is Phyllis.
The full name for Sue is Susan.
The full name for Liz is Elizabeth.
The full name for Maggie is Margaret.

Many famous people have been given nicknames:
Who was Farmer George? George III.
Who was the Virgin Queen? Elizabeth I.
Who was the Maid of Orleans? Joan of Arc.
Who was the Merrie Monarch? Charles II.
Who was the Iron Chancellor? Bismarck.
Who was the Iron Duke? Wellington.
Who was called Boney? Napoleon.
Who was called Dizzy? Benjamin Disraeli.
Finally, who was the Grand Old Lady of Threadneedle Street? The Bank of England.
Did you have a nickname at school or work?

Here are a few more everyday expressions using name:
I'm interested in buying your car — *name a price*.
Why, in the *name of commonsense*, did you do it? (Such interpolated phrases are difficult for a lipreader, who cannot read commas.)

Why, in the *name of goodness*, did you let her have it?
He has a *name for honesty* and good living.
Someone, who shall be *nameless*, has gone off with the towel.

We remarked earlier that *b* was similar to *m*. As we are talking about names, let us see how the teddybear received its name and look at the shape for b as in bear/bare.

The teddybear was named after President Theodore Roosevelt. While he was on a hunting expedition in the Rocky Mountains he adopted a bear as a pet. A bright business man in Brooklyn began to manufacture toy bears. He wrote to the President for permission to use his name, Teddy. Roosevelt replied, 'I don't think my name is likely to be worth much in the bear business but you are welcome to use it.'

Since then more than 150 million teddybears have been sold all over the world.

Repetition
Look for p, b, m.

Some people cannot bear to watch a violent film.
Some people cannot bear to see a person begging in the street.
Some people cannot bear to hear the details of someone's operation.
Some people cannot bear to watch acrobats high above the circus ring.
Some people cannot bear to see food wasted and thrown into the dustbin.
Some people cannot bear to part with their money.
Some people cannot bear to walk about with bare feet.

Here is a progressive sentence. It would be good practice if the helper read the first phrase, went back to the beginning, and then added the next and so on, to give the lipreader a chance to look at words starting and ending with b, and with b in the middle.

I'd like to throw this old *book* in the ru*bb*ish/*b*ecause it's falling apart/*b*ut my hus*b*and likes it/and I don't want to ru*b* him up the wrong way.

Drill: I'll rub it off,
        I'll rub it out,

      I'll rub it away,
      I'll rub it in.

The final three words have a definite rhythm with the 'it' being invisible to the lipreader.

Because is a common word that can appear in any part of a sentence.
    At the start — I was meeting a friend outside the theatre.

Because I was early — I went in and bought the tickets.
Because I was early — I had time for a drink.
Because I was early — I walked round the block.
Because I was early — I went and bought some chocolates.
    In the middle —
I put on a headscarf because it was windy.
I put on a raincoat because it was raining hard.
I put on a furcoat because it was freezing outside.
I put on an overcoat because the weather had turned chilly.
    Occasionally people will shrug and say, 'I'm doing it just because . . .' and leave the sentence unfinished.

As for p, it is such a good shape to see that it would be more profitable to look at some of the problems that specific words cause and then look at p's similarity to b/m.
    The little word 'up', which is only a p shape to the lipreader, is used in everyday language almost more than any other two-letter word. We attach it, quite unnecessarily most of the time, to verbs and it becomes incorporated into the verb for the lipreader.
    We polish up the silver.
    We light up a cigarette.
    We lock up the house.
    We fix up the car.
    We line up for tickets.
    We dress up for an occasion.
    We open up a shop in the morning and shut it up at night.
    We think up excuses.
    We work up an appetite.
    We fill up a hot water bottle.
    If you are up to it you can try making a list of the ways in which 'up' is used. It will take up a lot of your time but if you don't give up you will wind up with several thousands!

Difficult phrases are — If I feel up to it.
It's up to you.
He's all up the creek.
It's all up in the air.

You will see that there are several little words coming together and some, like 'it' are lost on the mouth. It is worthwhile taking these occasionally for both watching and listening practice and then incorporating them into sentences. For example:

I'll be there tomorrow if I feel up to it.
If I feel up to it I'll be there tomorrow.
I don't mind what we do, it's up to you.
It's up to you what we do, I don't mind.
I don't know that he's supposed to be doing, he's all up the creek.
He's all up the creek, I don't know what he's supposed to be doing.
Nobody has made any plans, it's all up in the air.
It's all up in the air, nobody has made any plans.

Lipreaders rarely have the chance to enjoy a joke. Sometimes they manage to read most of the story, only to miss out on the punchline and then they find the narrator is not prepared to repeat this because everyone else is laughing. From the speaker's viewpoint, a joke loses in the second telling and for the lipreader it has been a wasted effort. For this reason it is a change to be able to read one from your helper. The following contains plenty of p b and m shapes.

Solomon Levy wanted to buy his wife a present for her birthday.

'What would you like for your birthday, my dear?' he said. 'Would you like a mink coat, a string of pearls or a more modern car?'

'Oh Solomon,' said his wife, 'What would I be wanting with another mink coat, or a string of pearls or a more modern car. Buy me a plot in the cemetery, a nice piece of ground under the trees and I shall be happy.'

So Solomon bought her a green plot under the trees and she was very happy.

One year passed and this time Solomon did not mention birthdays. His wife waited all morning and then all afternoon, but in the evening she could wait no longer. 'Solomon,' she said, 'What are you going to give me for my birthday, this year?' 'Nothing,' he said crossly, 'because you haven't used last year's present yet.'

Still on p and b, put/book look very similar on the lips, although you may be able to hear the difference.
Try — I don't know where to put it down.
        I don't know where to book it down.

In this sentence of course the sense will tell you which is which —
    You can't find it! But I put the book where you'd be sure to see it.

If put is followed by 'it' you will have to look for the following word:
    I told her to put it down.
    I told her to put it off.
    I told her to put it back.
    I told her to put it forward.

Sometimes another word will follow 'put' —
    I said, 'I don't know why you *put up* with it'.
    I said, 'I don't know why you are so *put out*'.
    I said, 'I don't know why you *put in* so much time at your job'.
    I said, 'I don't know why you *put by* so little of your salary'.

Listen or lipread
Mr Butcher found the monthly management meetings rather *off-putting*. There was always a great deal of talk about *output* and *input*. Each manager *put forward* new proposals or tried to *put in* a good word for certain employees. Some of the ideas were extremely *well put* but they always had to *put up with* the few who tried to *put through* ridiculous notions and who were badly *put out* when told these were unacceptable.

Imaginative — give an answer
Where would you put these things to keep them fresh or safe?
Where would you put a sack of potatoes?
Where would you put a cheque for £100?

Where would you put a wet umbrella?
Where would you put a frozen shoulder of lamb?
Where would you put a book of stamps?
Where would you put a spare can of petrol?
Where would you put a box of hearing aid batteries?
Where would you put a spare pair of tights?
Where would you put an extra bottle of milk?

Since we said that some words starting with p, b, or m, will make similar shapes here is one short piece to show that very often it is a matter of the context solving the problem. Certainly pill/bill/mill are alike to a lipreader in isolation, whereas very often in language there is no confusion.

If you have a bottle of *pills* the label might say:
Take one pill before each meal.
Take one pill before retiring.
Take one pill after each meal.
Take one pill morning and evening.

People take sleeping pills to help them sleep.
People take slimming pills to help them lose weight.
People take pep pills to give themselves energy.
People take vitamin pills to make up deficiencies in their diet.
People take headache pills to relieve a pain in the head.
People take antibiotic pills to counteract a fever.

We all have a number of *bills* to pay each month.
We have bills for the electricity we have used.
We have bills for the gas we have burned.
We have bills for the food we have bought.
We have bills for the rates we have to pay.
We have bills for the repairs to our car.
We have bills for the water we use.
We have bills for the jobs the odd-job man has done for us.

What is the largest *bill* you have to pay?

Mr Miller has many problems. His wife recently went off and left him for another man. He works for an evening paper and may be made redundant at work. He is a compulsive gambler and has lost a lot of money betting on the horses. Last week his beautiful new Morris was stolen. The police found the car but the radio had been ripped out, the wipers were missing, the battery was flat and there was no petrol left in it. You might say that he is going through the *mill*.

And here is something to stretch the more advanced lipreaders. It can be used for involvement, or as a game.

In the Bible we have many books — here are some clues for a few of the well-known sections of the Bible.
This book is for men who preside in courts of law (Judges).
This book means the start of something (Genesis).
This book has given us many wise sayings (Proverbs).
This book is like sections of a play (Acts).
This book is only partly warm (Luke).
This book is a very poor comforter (Job).
This book is full of grief and woe (Lamentations).
This book brings bad luck (Jonah).
This book is useful for mathematicians (Numbers).
This book has a girl's name (Ruth).
This book is full of sacred songs (Psalms).
This book is one piece of German money (Mark).
This book means a going out (Exodus).

Drill: Look for the word 'book'. Which sentence is the helper saying?
Have you read this book?
Have you finished with this book?
What did you think of that book?
What book are you reading?

Imaginative clueing for lipreading.
Mr Brown was trying out his new car. He went down the M1 at over 100 m.p.h. He was eventually booked for speeding.

We wanted to do something different on our wedding anniversary. My husband would have taken me to a dance but I said I would rather he booked for the theatre as I enjoy a good play.

I had a terrible journey last weekend. I thought the train would be more or less empty but it was full of football crowds so I wished afterwards that I had booked a seat.

Involvement —
What book would you choose to take on a cruise?
What book would you choose if you were holidaying on a remote island?

What book would you choose to read on the train?
What book would you choose to carry around in your pocket?
What book would you choose to give to your wife on her next birthday?
What book would you choose if you were sent to prison?
What book would you choose for a long spell in hospital?
What book would you choose to read in a foreign country?
What book would you choose as a Christmas present for a maiden aunt?
What book would you choose while waiting at an airport?

Listening practice
We are so used to seeing books as *pages of print* between hard or *soft covers* that we forget a book may *come in many* shapes and *guises*.

Many publishers have tried different ways of *altering type* to catch public attention. You may remember the page in *Alice in Wonderland* where the piece called the Mouse's Tale *zigzags* down the page in smaller and smaller type. There is a book called *The Machine* which is bound in *metal*. It is riveted down the *spine* and the *dust* jacket is *hinged on*. It is a book on engineering. There is a book called *All my Chairs* which comes in a *sack tied with string*. Each chapter is a roll of *cloth* printed with chair *designs*. There are no words. A Mr Johnson has written a book with *twenty-seven loose* chapters. The reader *shuffles these like* a pack of cards and reads *in any* order he likes. But the world's *heaviest* book *is said to* be the Apocalypse. The cover of this book is *designed* by Salvador Dali. The book weighs 460 lb *and is* worth a million dollars because the cover *consists* of emeralds, agates, *bronze*, *knives*, forks and 585 nails.

The words and phrases in italics (apart from book titles) would be difficult for those with high frequency deafness but, as in lipreading, can be guessed at with a mental effort, so repeat and give 'thinking' time.

I remember, in my teens, having a book which I kept for autographs. These books are called albums (Latin albus = white) as they are unprinted books for making collections of something. *Repetition of a phrase:*

I remember having a stamp album.
I remember having a postcard album.
I remember having a photograph album.
I remember having an album of cigarette cards.
I remember having an album of pressed flowers.
I remember having an autograph album.

I passed the autograph album round to my friends and they all wrote something in it.

One popular line was — By hook or by crook I'll be last/first in this book. This was always written on one of the flyleafs. Now look at the following and use them for lipreading practice.

I wish you health I wish you wealth
I wish you golden store
I wish you Heaven after Death
What can I wish you more?

and,

Through this and every coming year
May happiness reign o'er you
Around your path may joy appear
And sunshine go before you.

Well I shall be 'brought to book' if I go on about books any more. But before we stop have another look at the drill — and try to get these first time.

Repeat: What did you think of that book?
Have you finished with this book?
Have you read this book?
What book are you reading?

Jaw Movements

The advanced reader should be watching how a jaw movement changes the rhythm of words. Each time we utter a fresh syllable we make a jaw movement and sometimes this is the only indication that two words are unlike.

Look at — pick, picnic, and Piccadilly, where the only truly visible shape is the initial consonant p, just to see the jaw move up and down.

But a phrase can help with meaning:

It was left to me to *pick up the pieces*.
I do wish he wouldn't *pick at his food*.

He *will pick fault* with everything I do.
She's only come to *pick my brains*.

A picnic

Sometimes food tastes better out of doors. In the days of
Mrs Beeton, people made a great occasion of a picnic. In her
book she tells of all the articles which are necessary and
which should not be forgotten at a picnic. Here are some of
the essentials in her view: you should pack (not pick) a
bottle of mint sauce well corked, good oil and pounded
sugar, a stick of horseradish, made mustard. If it can be
managed, take a little ice. It is hardly necessary to say that
plates, tumblers, wine glasses, knives, forks and spoons
must not be forgotten. Also teacups and saucers, three or
four teapots, some lump sugar and milk. Take three
corkscrews.

That all sounds very practical advice but what usually
happens at a picnic?

The wasps come and settle on the jam.
The bees come and settle on the honey.
The flies come and settle on everything.
The cows come and look over your shoulder.
The tablecloth flies away from its anchorage.
The butter melts before you can use it.
The milk spills.
The children run about with food in their hands.
The grass you've chosen is the most prickly in the
neighbourhood.
The ground is the most uneven.
The farmer is the most unfriendly.
And just when everyone is ready to eat the clouds open.
In other words it's no picnic to go on a picnic!

Words with different shapes

It is helpful to concentrate on a few words with very
different shapes and then see these used in a context.

For example — look at, went, saw, felt, heard, smelled,
ate. Now look for them in the following short pieces. They
will be in order. Attempt one or two at a time.

I went to Woolworths. I saw a friend there. I felt her
touch me on the shoulder. I heard a lot of gossip from her. I
smelled all the food as we talked in the shop. We stayed and
ate a sandwich there.

I went to the cinema. I saw a new film. I felt disappointed with it. I heard people shuffling their feet behind me. I smelled someone's pipe. I ate some peanuts in the interval.

I went to the park. I saw the lilies opening on the pond. I felt sleepy. While I sat on the grass I heard the children playing. I smelled the roses. I ate the sandwiches I'd brought with me.

I went to the market. I saw all the stalls. I felt very excited. I heard all the dealers shouting their wares. I smelled the fruit and vegetables they were selling. I ate one of the apples I bought.

I went into the chemist's. I saw my neighbour there. I felt sorry for her, she has been so ill. I heard her call me. I smelled the horrid medicine she has to take. I ate a throat lozenge she gave me.

Lipreading Practice with Nursery Rhymes

The next few lessons are based on nursery rhymes. There is nothing shaming about using such rhymes with adults, if one is going to use the language as lesson material in a practical way. Adults have the learned rhythm of these rhymes in the deep cortex of their brains and I have found sometimes that if I tap out the lines of a rhyme with a cleaning rubber on a blackboard some will recognize the rhyme from the beat. Usually they are most interested in the historical event behind the rhyme and they enjoy recalling something they once knew extremely well, which, in fact, they have never really forgotten.

The helper should let the lipreader read the chosen rhyme, although in a class an effort would be made to ask students to make a guess. Usually first lines such as hickory, dickory dock are difficult, but the second line usually contains a clue and each rhyme has its own especial beat. After such lessons a class can become very adept at giving back the second line of any rhyme they have known well, and it is very good practice in quick response and the use of familiar language.

Hickory dickory dock
  Hickory dickory dock
  The mouse *ran up* the clock
  The clock *struck* one
  The mouse *ran down*
  Hickory dickory dock.

This rhyme must have been written after 1789, when Dr Guillotin invented his device for beheading prisoners.

We still use the word dock for the place where punishment is meted out and, of course, we dock a horse's tail. Hickory is a hard wood which was used to build the guillotine. Dickory comes from the word dicky meaning shaky, because the structure was not meant to be permanent. We still say people look dicky when they appear shaky and unfit.

The mouse refers to the blade as it scurried down after its prey and 'ran up the clock' is the blade being raised.

Down it ran has two meanings: first, the clock has run down and the prisoner's time has run out; and, secondly, the blade is on its way. So the last line means that the victim has been docked by the hickory dickory.

Let's look at stuck/struck/truck.

I was very struck by your last remark.

It suddenly struck me that we could cash in on his plan.

He was struck dumb/dumbstruck by the destruction he saw all round him.

He would have no truck with the proposal.

I can't finish the crossword, I'm stuck.

He struck gold/oil/it rich.

He was struck with amazement/terror/surprise/dismay.

I'm stuck for words/ideas/cash/with the job.

'Ran' is often followed by a positional word:

Ran up — I ran up the road to catch the milkman.

Ran down — I ran down the stairs two at a time.

Ran past — I ran past the shop before I realized I'd gone too far.

Ran in — I ran in the shop just as it was closing.

Ran out — I ran out to get another pint of milk.

Ran back — I ran back for my raincoat.

Ran forward — I ran forward to greet him as he stepped off the plane.

Ran for — I ran for my life.

Many women are afraid of mice but most of us have a *fear* or *pho*bia. Crime, drugs or drink are not the main hazards of life that we are sometimes led to expect. The average person is far more worried about other things, ordinary things like speaking before a group or being inside a lift. A team of researchers asked three thousand people what things they feared most. The table showed that: 41 per cent were afraid of speaking before a group of people; 32 per cent were afraid of heights; 22 per cent were afraid of spiders and other insects; 22 per cent were afraid of deep water and flying; 14 per cent were afraid of loneliness; 8 per cent were afraid of the dark; 8 per cent were afraid of lifts; and 5 per cent were afraid of escalators.

These fears are so widespread that they must be regarded as normal. In general men were not as afraid of things as women, but perhaps they only said this to the researchers to appear braver than they really are.

Mary had a little lamb

Mary had a little lamb
It's feet were white as snow
And everywhere that Mary went
That lamb was sure to go.

These are said to be the best known four lines in the English language. The rhyme was first published in 1830 and written by a Mrs Sarah Hale who lived in Boston in Lincolnshire. She based it on an incident that was partly true. The Welsh claimed that a girl named Mary Hughes was the original Mary who appears in the verses and this appears on her tombstone. However, it is probable that the story of an adopted lamb going to school with a child has happened many times in the countryside.

'Sure to go' is a difficult phrase out of the context of the rhyme.

Practise these combinations of 'sure to':
Whatever we do it's sure to be wrong.
Whatever I do, I'm sure to make a mistake.
Whatever he does, it's sure to be right.
Whatever she does, she's sure to please him.

There are a few modern additions to the nursery rhyme — can you lipread them?
Mary had a little lamb
Her father shot it dead
And now it goes to school with her
Between two hunks of bread.

and
  Mary had a little lamb
  It was a greedy glutton
  She fed it ice cream every day
  And now it's frozen mutton.

Half a pound of tuppeny rice
  Half a pound of *tuppeny* rice
  Half a pound of *treacle*
  Mix it up and make it nice
  Pop goes the weasel.

  Up and down the City Road
  In and out the Eagle
  That's the way the money goes
  Pop goes the weasel.

A weasel was used in the tailoring trade — it is the name for the pressing iron. When trade was bad and there was no money to buy rice and treacle, the tailor would pawn his iron in the pop shop.

A large number of small tailor shops were in the City Road and the Eagle was the pub where they went and met for their beer. So that was another way the money went and another reason for popping or pawning the iron.

Two pence would buy you very little these days.
In 1926 2p would have bought you: 2 boxes of matches, a newspaper, 2 postcards, 2 platform tickets, a large ice cream and a ride from the Bank to King's Cross (and back).

Treacle is an interesting word, from the Greek meaning *antidote*. Treacle was used by the Romans as a medicine and we know the Greeks used it in the same way, as well as to dress wounds.

The words treacle and real look alike to the lipreader:
  I don't believe it's real/treacle.

Treacle is full of minerals — you can spread treacle on bread.
                                  you can melt it over a pudding.
                                  you can eat it from a spoon.
                                  you can beat it into milk for a bedtime drink.

> you can boil it to make treacle toffee.
>
> you can smear it on a cut or a graze.

Whichever way you use it, treacle is good for you.

Half a moment — I'd like a word with you.

She doesn't *half* go on/half think she's somebody/someone.

This one is better by *half*.

The workforce has been cut by more than *half*.

Pop game:

This pop is licked by children (lollipop).

This pop is a flower (poppy).

This pop is a noisy toy (pop gun).

This pop is a little darling (poppet).

This pop is a character from a film (Mary Poppins or Popeye).

This pop is a relative (Grandpop).

This pop is a vegetable (popcorn).

Iron:

We must *iron out* our differences.

I'm just going to do some ironing.

I've a pile of ironing to do.

The old weasel was a heavy pressing iron made of cast iron. These irons have gone out of fashion but are often used as a doorstop/used to press meat/used to press flowers in the leaves of a book.

Nowadays we can buy an electric iron, a steam iron, or an automatic iron.

Odd Words

There are odd words used in language that get in the way but don't add meaning and yet the lipreader must realize they are there.

Yet is one such word — 'Haven't you finished yet?' The lipreader will see movement after 'finished' but has read the sense so can ignore the last word.

Quite is another such word and may be a bother since it starts with the same shape as w and may be read as something else.

For practice — I haven't quite finished.
I haven't quite made up my mind.
I haven't quite decided.
I haven't quite got enough.
I haven't quite had enough.

Got is another horror
Have you got a pen?
Have you got a headache?
Have you got a spare minute?
Have you got a moment to spare?
Have you got a cold?
Have you got a spare battery?

Just is particularly poor to read as it is often in conjunction with another lipreadable word, e.g. just going or just isn't. It is easiest when it ends a sentence as the following practice will show.

Repetition
Don't wait for me — I'm just going to finish this letter.
Don't wait for me — I'm just going to leave a note for the milkman.
Don't wait for me — I'm just going to give the cat its fish.

Turn these round
I'm just going to finish this letter — don't wait for me.
I'm just going to leave a note for the milkman — don't wait for me.
I'm just going to give the cat its fish — don't wait for me.
    Would expression and voice tone help? Try to lipread these and then listen to them.

It just isn't right! It just isn't fair! It just doesn't make sense! It just isn't so.

Now read it at the end of a sentence.
    When I left you last night I caught the last bus — but only just.
    When I left you last night I got home before my wife — but only just.
    When I left you I reached home before the rain started — but only just.
    Just let me tell you a little story I've *just read*. An old lady was sitting in a railway carriage. The train was *just about* to

start when a young man jumped in. He sat opposite the old lady and *just kept* chewing a stick of gum. The old lady watched him steadily for a few minutes, then she leaned across and *just tapped* him on the leg. 'Excuse me *just a minute*,' she said, 'I am *just a little* hard of hearing and I'm not a very good lipreader so I *just don't* know a word you've said to me.'

> Just a minute — you've left your pen behind.
>   — I wanted a word with you.
>   — I haven't finished what I wanted to say.
>   — I want to see whether I've forgotten anything.
>   — don't be in such a hurry.

And you might have to lipread, in the legal sense, someone remarking 'That was just'.

These small words are part of a sentence and do have a grammatical place but, for the lipreader, it is more important to recognize the subject matter, the nouns, and the verbs which will convey the gist of what someone is speaking about. For this reason I believe it important to practise the familiar phrases used in speech, so that the essential shapes are picked out from the rhythm of the whole.

For example, using the common phrase, 'Isn't it . . .' will help the lipreader to let it go, hang on and wait for the first words that have shape.

Isn't it a funny thing about George and Margaret — *who'd have thought* they'd have split up?

Isn't it a hoot about Mary — *who'd have thought* she'd apply for that job?

Isn't it strange about Robert — *who'd have thought* he'd have given up such a good post?

Isn't it peculiar about Sarah — *who'd have thought* she would react like that?

Isn't it a good thing we brought our raincoats — *we'd have been* soaked in this storm.

Isn't it a good thing we like spaghetti — *we'd have gone* hungry otherwise in Rome.

Isn't it a good thing we brought our cheque books — *we couldn't* have bought much without them.

Hymns for Practice

I have had a client who had lessons from many teachers of lipreading during the twenty years she was deaf. Her first remark to me was, 'I want no schoolboy howlers and no Bible stories!' Certainly plays on words are often lost on lipreaders and Bible stories need refashioning for modern speech. However, I have found that some of the stories behind well-known hymns lend themselves to useful practice.

The lipreader needs to read the verse of the hymn first. One method of continuing is to give the reader the piece to be lipread with some of the phrases left out, so that he has the gist of the story, but it can just as easily be done, if he is advanced, by lipreading the whole. (But remember that the lipreader does not lipread the verse — there would be no point since the language is archaic.)

Example: Rock of Ages, cleft for me
Let me hide myself in thee.
Let the water and the blood
From thy riven side which flowed
Be of sin the double cure
Cleanse me from its guilt and power.
(by Augustus Montague Toplady)

This gentleman with the illustrious name was born in Surrey in 1740. Later he became a preacher and was sent to a parish in the West Country. One day he was walking in the hills when he was caught in a thunderstorm. It was so savage that he had to find shelter. The rain lashed down and the lightning zigzagged among the clifftops. Then he saw a cleft in the rocks. He ran towards it and found he could just stand upright in it. When he reached home he composed this hymn, implying that he was seeking sanctuary in God. The hymn was published in 1775 and became an established favourite. It has been sung in missions, on board ships, and even at Wembley on Cup Final Day. Pilgrims still go to the cleft in the rock on the last Saturday in July and sing the great hymn outside the cleft.

Cleft/left will look alike on the lips since the sound of k is a back consonant.

Cleft is uncommon unless one is remarking that a person has a cleft palate or a cleft in his chin.

The *left-hand side* has always been the sinister or evil side.

Men's clothes button from *left to right*, presumably to leave their sword arm free.

If a person is clumsy they are told that they have *two left feet*.

Left is also used with a positional word, making a short phrase with its own rhythm. For example:

I *left before* she did.
I *left after* she did.
I *left out* the most important part.
I *left in* high spirits.
I *left on* the 12.30 from Victoria.
I *left off* my coat, it was such a warm day.
I *left through* the main door.
I *left by* the back door.
I *left down* the back stairs.
I *left under* a cloud.
I *left behind* my keys and purse.
I *left for* the last time.
I *left just* in time.

Imaginative — give an answer. The helper should produce the following few articles and ask the appropriate questions.

This handkerchief was *left behind* on my armchair — who could my visitor have been?

This piece of flex was *left on* my kitchen sink — who could the workman have been?

This piece of old bone was *left by* the back door — what animal could have *left it* there?

This circular was *left for me* to read — who could the caller have been?

Look at the difference a good visible consonant can make to a word — let, left.

Which one is your helper saying? I just let it.
                                              I just left it.

He left out the most important part.
He let out the most important part.

Visual Clues in Practice

While speaking of showing things, a visual clue (as above) is most helpful to stir up the imagination. Here is some practice work using a few *common objects*.

This is a handkerchief (helper holds it out) and then repeats the difficult introductory phrase before using the list:

You can use a handkerchief as a bandage.

You can use a handkerchief to wrap your lunch in.

You can use a handkerchief to wipe your shoes.

You can use a handkerchief as a reminder by tying a knot in one corner.

You can use a handkerchief as a head cover in hot weather.

You can use a handkerchief as a duster.

You can use a handkerchief to grace your breast pocket.

You can also use a handkerchief to blow your nose!

This is a hairpin:

You can use a hairpin to pick a lock.

You can use a hairpin to prise out a winkle.

You can use a hairpin to pick your teeth.

You can use a hairpin to scratch a name on wood.

You can use a hairpin to lever a battery from your hearing aid.

You can use a hairpin to clean out your ear mould.

You can use a hairpin to dig out the bits of a walnut.

You can also use a hairpin to fasten your hair.

This is a piece of cardboard:

You can use a piece of cardboard to leave a note for the milkman.

You can use a piece of cardboard to stop a table from wobbling.

You can use a piece of cardboard to wedge a door open.

You can use a piece of cardboard to make a laundry list.

You can use a piece of cardboard to make a bingo card.

You can use a piece of cardboard to make a template.

You can also use a piece of cardboard to make a notice.

Using Imagination

Another imaginative exercise is to lipread a short experience in everyday terms. The helper can just give the lipreader the introductory phrase as a clue.

On my way home last night — I bought the evening paper.

On my way home last night — I collected a suit from the cleaners.

On my way home last night — I waited half an hour for a bus.

On my way home last night — I met an old friend on the bus.

On my way home last night — I bought some fish and chips to take home for supper.

On my way to the theatre — I took the tube to Leicester Square.

On my way to the theatre — I bought a box of chocolates.

On my way to the theatre — I had a drink in a bar.

On my way to the theatre — I bought a paper.

On my way to the theatre — I met my friend on the corner of the square.

Then to bring in some well-known names and places.

If I visited the Tower of London I might see — the Crown jewels.

If I visited the Tower of London I might see — the ravens on the lawn.

If I visited the Tower of London I might see — the Beefeaters.

If I visited the Tower of London I might see — the Bloody Tower.

If I visited the Tower of London I might see — the dungeons.

If I visited the Tower of London I might see — the room where the two princes were murdered.

If I visited Buckingham Palace I might see — the changing of the guard.

If I visited Buckingham Palace I might see — the Royal coach and horses.

If I visited Buckingham Palace I might see — the Queen's Gallery.

If I visited Buckingham Palace I might see — the statue of Queen Victoria.

If I visited Buckingham Palace I might see — the royal emblem flying.

If I visited Buckingham Palace I might see — hundreds of tourists.

If I visited Parliament Square — I'd see the Houses of Parliament.

If I visited Parliament Square — I'd see Big Ben.

If I visited Parliament Square — I'd see Westminster Abbey.

If I visited Parliament Square — I'd see some statues of famous men.

If I visited Parliament Square — I'd see flags of all nations.

If I visited Parliament Square — I'd see fleets of buses.

Non-visible Words

I found it useful, when the lipreader had attained some skill, to be able to show that although many words were not visible on the lips, and in isolation, when attached to another word or phrase they became decipherable. Here are a few lessons to illustrate this point; it seems more profitable to do this than to give work on visible shapes.

Good is a word in point — no wonder the born deaf need a sign for it. Yet with another clue it is not thought of as an invisible or poor shape.

Drill:

Good afternoon.
Good grief.
Good gracious.
Goodness me.
My goodness.

It's no good is little better. Repeat:

It's no good — I can't make him see reason.
It's no good — I can't make him see sense.
It's no good — I can't get this top off.
It's no good — I haven't the money to go abroad this year.

I've looked at your proposition carefully, but it's no good.
I've thought over all you said, but it's no good.
I've found a cheaper make, but it's no good.

Mr Jeffreys owned a very good business. He was in good health and had good cause to feel satisfied.

Harry's idea of a good time was to have plenty of good fun.

Mary was a good sort. Many people had good reason to be glad they knew her. She was full of goodwill and would always have a good try at helping others.

What makes a good holiday — sea, sun and good food.

What makes a good book — the plot, the writing and the characters.

What makes a good meal — the food, the company and a good wine.

What makes a good film — the acting, the cast, and the story.

What makes a good concert — the hall, the orchestra, and the pieces to be played.

What makes a good plan — simplicity, forethought and direction.

What makes a good lipreader — practice, quick thinking, and perseverence.

Another word that is unlipreadable — did.

Drill:
Did you?
Did they?
Did we?
Did she?

I do not recommend 'did I' or 'did he' because there is no good vowel shape to distinguish.

I was wondering if you'd posted the letter — did you?
I was wondering if they'd moved — did they?
I was wondering if we'd paid the rates — did we?
I was wondering if she's passed her exams — did she?

Did you post my letter?
Did they move?
Did we pay the rates?
Did she pass her exams?

What did the doctor say to you? 'Oh,' he said, 'Did I smoke a lot?'

What did the manager say to you? 'Oh,' he said, 'Did I

realize there is no chance of promotion at the moment?'

What did the headmaster say to you? 'Oh,' he said, 'Did I realize that my boy is brilliant at maths?'

What did the policeman say to you? 'Oh,' he said, 'Did I know that my car was on a yellow line?'

What did the ticket collector say to you? 'Oh', he said, 'Did I realize that my season expired last week?'

Responses

What did Raleigh do when he saw Queen Elizabeth stepping out into the rain?

What did Shakespeare leave to his wife in his Will?

What did Francis Drake do when the Armada came to attack England?

What did Joan of Arc do to help her country?

And in the world of fiction:

What did Aladdin do to summon the genie?

What did the spider do to Miss Muffet?

What did Jack Horner do?

What did Tom the piper's son steal?

What did Little Bo peep lose?

What did Old King Cole send for?

What did the Old Woman do to all her children?

How did you do that?

I broke my arm last week. How did you do that? I fell off a chair.

I crashed my car. How did you do that? Some fool came out of a side turning without stopping.

I lost my bag. How did you do that? I put it down on the counter and someone went off with it.

I won some money. How did you do that? I had 24 points on the football coupon.

I didn't want to go to the party last weekend but I didn't like to refuse. They did ask me last year and I did manage to find an excuse but this year I did think I should go. I didn't expect to enjoy it half as much as I did.

Did up: He did up the house before he sold it. She did up her coat before she went out in the cold.

Did for: Think of all he did for her!

Did hope: I did hope you'd be able to join us.

Did this: She did this before she went away.

Did that: She did that before she went away.
Did very well: They did very well in their exams.

What did you do last weekend/last night/before you came to class this evening/before you retired/when you left school/after you left school/for your holiday last year/last Christmas?

Case is another unlipreadable word.

At the start of a sentence it has to be slid over for a following clue:

In case we miss each other, I'll stand under the clock inside the station.

In case it rains, you had better put your mac in your bag.

In case there's a train strike I'll use the car to go to town tomorrow.

In the middle you may get clues either side:

I'd better buy another loaf in case we have visitors this weekend.

Let's take our cheque books in case we see something we'd like to buy.

I'll take an umbrella in case it rains.

I'll take a book in case we have a long wait at the station.

I'll take a flask of coffee in case there's nowhere to buy a drink.

At the end of a sentence:

I'll take an umbrella, in case. ('I need it' is understood.)

I'll take your telephone number, in case.

I'll take my cheque book, in case.

I'll take a spare pair of shoes, in case.

Involvement

Tell me three things you could put into a suitcase,

— three things you could put into a briefcase,

— something you could put down on a staircase,

— three things you could find in a needlecase,

— three things you could find in a pencil case,

— three things you could find in a writing case.

Imaginative

Here's a very strange case. A man was referred to a hospital in Leamington Spa. For a long time he had been complaining of stomach pains. His own doctor didn't know what to make of the case because there appeared nothing radically wrong. The man went to hospital for x-rays and it was found that his stomach was full of unexpected objects. He was operated on and from his stomach the surgeon took six one-inch nails, a ball of feathers, a small compass and four and a half pence in coins! Wasn't that an unusual case!

Recall
Remember we mentioned — a briefcase
                     — a needlecase
                     — a suitcase
                     — a pencil case.

As soon as you have sufficient clues tell me the case I am filling.
(The helper repeats each section, adding on an extra phrase each time to see whether the lipreader can name the case before he has all the clues.)

I'm filling a case with a ruler.
I'm filling a case with a ruler and a rubber.
I'm filling a case with a ruler and a rubber and some lead pencils. Which case am I filling?

I'm filling a case with underwear.
I'm filling a case with underwear and clothes.
I'm filling a case with underwear, clothes and shoes. Which case am I filling?

I'm filling a case with needles.
I'm filling a case with needles and pins.
I'm filling a case with needles and pins and a crochet hook. Which case am I filling?

(This last one is especially difficult since neither needles nor pins have much shape. Do not go on repeating the first two lines but tell the lipreader to wait until he has the last clue and then it is possible he will guess correctly.)

I'm filling a case with documents.
I'm filling a case with documents and a fountain pen.
I'm filling a case with documents, a fountain pen and some red tape.

Sometimes a phrase has three unlipreadable words together, for example 'in any case' and 'isn't the case' and 'in case I'.

Practise

In any case, we can compare notes later.

In any case, the weather is bound to be warm in July.

In any case, I shall be seeing you again next month.

I thought he had been here before, but that isn't the case.

I thought he had family living here, but that isn't the case.

I thought she went into hospital for a minor operation, but that isn't the case.

In case I don't see you, have a lovely holiday.

In case I don't have time, let someone else read it first.

In case the train is late, I'll meet you at the hotel.

In case we miss each other we had better have our own tickets.

Here is another rather amusing case:

Mrs Lawrence had been out shopping and stopped to have a cup of tea. As she was leaving the café she tripped over the step and broke her ankle. The proprietor rushed forward to help her when he saw her fall. He caught his elbow on a pot of boiling water which sent it pouring over his arm. Across the road a holidaymaker had been looking out of a window opposite the café. He saw Mrs Lawrence fall and raced down his stairs to help her, but he fell and broke his leg. So that when the ambulance arrived it took away three casualties — a woman with a broken ankle, a man with a scalded arm, and a man with a broken leg — what a chapter of accidents.

Remember, in case you are thinking of holidays:
    If you're packing a case for a holiday in Britain don't forget a raincoat.
    — in Majorca don't forget the suntan lotion.
    — in Warsaw don't forget a bar of soap. (Soap is rationed in Poland.)
    — in Moscow don't forget a pack of toilet paper. (Not all hotels supply it out there.)
    — in Morocco don't forget a tube of insect repellant.
    — in Greece don't forget a tin of dried milk. (The coffee is always black out there.)

Empty

This word could be written M.T. So we would see the name of these two letters if someone said, 'Let's empty the teapot' or, 'The teapot's empty'. In lipreading we need to lipread the names of letters at times, rather than the sound they make, because many abbreviations are used in speech. For example:

He gave me his I.O.U. and *I owe you* a fiver.

His car broke down on the M.1 and he sent for the A.A.

Did you watch BBC1 last night or ITV?

We reported the owner of the dog to the RSPCA.

Occasionally the abbreviation is pronounced as a word, for example, 'He works for UNO,' or, 'He works for the NAAFI'. Or you might hear, 'He works for You-Know-Who'.

These two sentences have different meanings and would be said in different voice tone: He works for who? He works for WHO. (World Health Organisation)

Tales of Nasreddin

In Persian folklore there is a Wise Man named Nasreddin. He has a store of little tales which make useful introductions to lipreading practice. They are not moral issues like Aesop's fables, and in some Nasreddin cuts rather a stupid figure, but they are amusing and often instructive. The following is one of the shorter examples.

Nasreddin went into a teahouse and said to all his friends, 'The Moon is much more useful than the Sun.'

'Why?' asked all his friends.

'Well,' replied Nasreddin, 'we need the light more during the night then we do during the daytime.'

Let us take the phrase he uses, *'much more useful'*.

I find my old kitchen knife *much more useful* than a potato peeler.

They decided it would be *much more useful* to split the house into three separate flats.

A hammer is *much more useful* than a piece of wood for knocking in a nail.

Here are two more Nasreddin tales which are simple enough to be read by beginners. The first shows that, although there is no difference in two words when one has the prefix ad- attached (vice, advice), the context helps sort out meaning.

Nasreddin was a Wise Man. One day he was sitting in a

café drinking coffee with his friends.

One friend said to Nasreddin, 'You are a wise man. Tell us, what do you think is the most valuable thing in the world?'

Nasreddin thought for a moment and then he replied, 'I think that the most valuable thing in the world is advice.'

'Then,' said another friend, 'What do you think is the least valuable thing in the world?'

Nasreddin thought for a moment and then he replied, 'I think that the least valuable thing in the world is advice.'

'How can that be?' said all his friends, 'How can advice be the most and the least valuable thing in the world?'

'Well,' replied Nasreddin. 'If you give someone advice and they take it, then it is the most valuable thing in the world. But if you give someone advice and they don't take it then it is the least valuable thing in the world.'

One day Nasreddin was walking through the countryside with a friend. He saw the cows chewing the grass and he saw the birds flying in the sky. He said to his friend, 'I wonder why Allah allowed the birds their freedom to fly and yet the poor cow is forced to remain with his feet firmly fixed upon the ground.' Just then a bird flew directly overhead and something wet plopped on to Nasreddin's hat.

Nasreddin took off his hat and looked at it and then said, 'Now I know why Allah, in his infinite wisdom, did not allow the cow to fly.'

Listening and Lipreading Practice
This exercise could profitably be used as listening practice since the combination 'ks' may be heard by hearing aid wearers.

X is not a sound we take singly in lipreading because it is really a combination of sounds — this makes it difficult for some people to hear as it is a combination of k/s in a word. Try saying tax/tacks and you will find that you are making the same shape and sound that you did for a word ending in ks.

Drill
Watch your helper say box — chocs — rocks — flocks (phlox) and see what happens at the end of these words.

There is a movement, although there will be no lip pattern.

Repetition

I've ordered a box for this evening. (For the theatre is understood.)

I've ordered a box of apples from the fruiterers for Christmas.

I've ordered a box of Coxes from the fruiterers for Christmas.

I've ordered a box of chocolates as a special treat for her birthday.

I've ordered a box of single flowers for the buttonholes.

I've ordered a box of stationery with our new address.

Imaginative

This is a longer piece, requiring a good strong voice.

The first person to put a picture on a chocolate box was Richard Cadbury. He painted his small daughter playing with her cat in 1868. He then thought it would be a good idea to have this printed on the lid of his firm's chocolate boxes.

The public liked the idea and today the choice is much the same — animals being number one, followed by babies, country views and flowers.

Even the shape of the box can affect sales. Oblong boxes are the first choice, then square, round and fancy boxes next.

If you buy a box with an adorable puppy on the lid, harden your heart when a four-footed friend begs for a chocolate from the box. Chocs are not recommended for dogs.

When the box is empty don't throw it away. *Box clever*. Fill it with dog biscuits and the chocolate smell will linger and make an ordinary biscuit more tempting for your pet.

Colloquial

Box and cox — this comes from a story about a woman who took in lodgers. She let a room to a Mr Box who worked in the daytime and the same room to a Mr Cox who worked at night. They used the room and the bed without knowing that another man shared the room! So if you play Box and Cox you shuffle about deceiving people.

Gilbert and Sullivan composed a light opera with this title.

Practical

It would be possible in the home to find several boxes containing different articles and use the phrase, 'This is a box of . . .' Alternatively fill one box with a variety of smaller items and use with the phrase, 'I've got a . . . in this box.'

Alternatively, use the word 'tax' in its various forms for further -ks practice.

Most things carry a tax these days. In the past the Government of the day has put a tax on strange things as a source of revenue. There has been a tax on the number of windows allowed in a house — so people filled in some of their windows.

There has been a tax on hats. Men's hats were allowed to be only a few inches high and taller hats carried a tax on them.

Nowadays we pay a tax on food, drink, transport, clothes, perfumes and cosmetics, furnishings, repair work — in fact it is difficult to think of anything that does not carry some form of tax. It is very taxing to have to work out how much tax is being put on all the things we buy. At least we do not have to tax our brains to work out our income tax, as the government does this for us.

Using Jokes

One means of making sure that a lipreader enjoys a joke is to use one at the start of a lesson and then extract the difficulties from it to use as practice material. Again, beginners should be allowed to read through the joke first. This does, of course, destroy all spontaneity and they then know the punchline, but it is asking a lot for someone to lipread and carry the meaning through to the end. A beginner is often so intent on following each phrase that his mind forgets what he has read several seconds previously. If the lipreader is wearing an aid then he could well listen to his helper and watch while she reads the joke clearly and steadily. The words in italics will prove to be difficulties and need to be worked on afterwards.

An *elderly* farmer married a *young* girl. The girl was very beautiful and *no one knew* why she had married him.

A few weeks after the wedding the farmer met the *vicar*. The farmer had a very long face and started *complaining* to the vicar, '*I can't get my work done*. My wife is so beautiful that I *can't keep my hands off* her.'

'Well,' said the vicar, 'my advice is to give it time.'

They met about a month later and the same conversation took place, so the vicar said, 'Well, *it's still early* days, give it a bit more time.'

When another month had passed they met once more and this time the farmer looked quite cheerful.
'Ah,' said the vicar, 'you're looking less worried — is it working out alright?'

'Yes, vicar,' replied the farmer, 'I *got rid of* all my hands and now I've got her all to myself.'

Points arising from the joke:
I got rid of it
I was turning out my gloryhole last weekend.
I found a teapot with a broken spout — so I got rid of it.
I found a broken radio — so I got rid of it.
I found a leaky hot water bottle — so I got rid of it.
I found a rusty biscuit tin — so I got rid of it.
I found a blanket with the moth in it — so I got rid of it.
I found a percolator without a lid — so I got rid of it.
I found an empty wine bottle — so I got rid of it.
I found a storage jar without a cork — so I got rid of it.
     Good riddance to bad rubbish!

Repetition
No one knew — anything about it.
              — what he was up to.
              — what to do about it.
              — where we were going.
              — what to make of it.
              — how we'd get home.
              — why he hadn't turned up.
              — when the next plane was due.
              — what was happening.

I can't get my work done — through worrying about him.
                      — because she keeps on talking.
                      — with all these interruptions.

Then in reverse:
     With all these interruptions I can't get my work done.
     Because she keeps on talking I can't get my work done.

Through worrying about him I can't get my work done.

Involvement
Hands:
Who hands out tickets at the station?
Which animal is measured in hands?
What is the end of this proverb — Many hands . . .
Who would shout, 'All hands on deck'?
Who reads fortunes from hands?
Who tells fortunes from hands?
Who carries handcuffs?
Finish this proverb — A bird in the hand . . .
What does this phrase mean — 'To go cap in hand'?
Who would lead a hand-to-mouth existence?
Who would you give a big hand to?
Just a moment — I must get a *hand*kerchief.
I keep a miscellaneous collection of oddments at the bottom of my *hand*bag.
This is a letter from my *elderly* aunt — she's written to say that the *Vicar* has just called on her.
This is an unfinished letter. I'm *complaining to the* Electricity Board about my latest bill.
Here are a few spare Biros. I like to keep some *in hand*.
This is a lucky horseshoe sent by a friend who got *married* recently.
Here are a few boiled sweets — I *hand* these round on a journey.

Here is another joke which, sadly, could well be true.
A man was talking about his new hearing aid.
'It's absolutely marvellous,' he said. 'I can hear a leaf drop at 100 yards, a drop of water sounds like an explosion, and I hear noises from the flat next door — it's the best hearing aid in the world.'
His friend said, 'What kind is it?'
The man replied, 'A quarter to nine.'

Drill
It's absolutely marvellous!
It's absolutely splendid!
It's absolutely horrifying!
It's absolutely disgusting!

The last word — disgusting — has the unlipreadable prefix, dis-. This presents no lip shape but, when included as part of the word, a jaw movement must be made. Look for a few moments at the following:

may/dismay
bar/disbar
close/disclose
appoint/disappoint

You will notice the movement for the syllable. This may well be difficult to see in running speech, or on a poor speaker, and then context must be the guide.

A few practice sentences:

Mother was given an apron for Christmas. She was very disappointed — she'd rather have had a bottle of exotic perfume.

Father was given a tie for Christmas. He was very disappointed — he would rather have had a Black and Decker tool kit.

Auntie was given a tea cosy for Christmas. She was very disappointed — she would rather have had a bottle of gin.

Granny was given a box of hankies for Christmas. She was very disappointed — she would rather have had a cashmere shawl.

Grandad was given a pipe for Christmas. He was very disappointed — he would rather have had a box of expensive cigars.

There are other invisible prefixes, which is why the born deaf have problems with meaning. Truth resembles untruth, legal resembles illegal, and regular resembles irregular, and in these cases the opposite meaning is made. It is not always possible to guess from context but when the lipreader has reached this stage of practice then he will have become either adept at making a sensible guess, confident enough to be able to ask for a repeat or change of language, or a great pretender, as all of us have to be at times when we are faced with unusual situations, new faces, and varying modes of speech.

Progress in Lipreading

It is difficult to devise any means of testing progress in lipreading skill. But a teacher may do this by producing graded material, stemming from the easier lipreadable language to more unreadable phrases. There are some old English riddles and verses which are usable with the more advanced, as long as the lipreader is primed to give back *exactly* what he believes he sees — in this way one is able to judge whether all phonemes are known and lipreaders appear to find enjoyment and gratification in getting these right.

I have tried the following type of exercise in which the lipreader has to lipread despite mental distraction. If, as an example, you say you are going to give wellknown proverbs but change the endings of each saying, then presumably their mind is tuned in to anticipate the ending they know. If I say, 'People who live in glass houses . . .' they would be primed to finish with, 'should never throw stones'. Yet if I give them a different ending they must concentrate on reading something unexpected by shape, overcoming the natural inclination to complete the proverb normally.

Try a few out:
People who live in glass houses — will feel very warm in summer.
An apple a day — is a starvation diet.
Many hands — make a very large horse.
Look after the pennies — and the government will look after the pounds.
While the cat's away — there's less fur on the carpets.
It's a long road — when you have very short legs.
There's no smoke — in a non-smoking compartment.
Too many cooks — make a mess of the kitchen.
A stitch in time — saves you bleeding to death.
Two heads — will make you a monster.
New brooms — cost a lot of money.

It can be useful to give two similar sentences and point out the small differences that a good lipreader must strive to see. Many depend on the rhythmic beat of the syllables, giving an extra jaw movement, others depend on seeing one visible consonant that does not appear in the contrasting sentence. Take two or three in a practice session and repeat several times, finally asking the lipreader, 'Which one is this?'.

He is a sorter at the Post Office.
His daughter is at the Post Office.

When do you leave?
Where do you live?

Tell me what I can do.
Tell me what happened to you.

I was out of town for some time.
I was down south for some time.

He stayed on the path.
He strayed from the path.

You're talking nonsense.
You've got a guilty conscience.

I bought a new book with the money.
I bought a new book with me.

I must buy a chicken.
I must pay the cheque in.

He was hardly conscious.
It's on my conscience.

Have you brought the car keys?
Have you brought the tickets?

I'm just going down to the village shop.
I'm just going down to the fish shop.

Quick Responses

In the early days of lipreading instruction all stress was on analysing speech, watching lip movements and connecting these with the form of sounds, hence the designation 'lipreading'. Then, as in all educational fields, a swing came in the opposite direction. Teachers grew bored with taking lessons on single shapes, or found it difficult to make interesting material from these week after week, and started to talk about 'running speech' and 'speech reading'. This enabled them to take colloquial language and, in fact, make lessons much more applicable to everyday life.

Ideally there is room for both. I have met extremely good lipreaders who, because of lack of knowledge of the theory of shapes, were not very good at making a quick mental switch when necessary. After a few weeks of basic sound shapes, their lipreading was even better.

But, more important even than these two modes of teaching, is the need to stimulate mental reaction. We say that the lipreader needs to make an intelligent guess, without doing very much to give practice on this essential factor.

So here are a few suggestions to help him towards a quick response. The lipreader follows the sentence and then tries to finish with his own words immediately the helper stops. At first it is usual for the reader to repeat what he has just read but with practice this step is left out and an immediate response is forthcoming. There will be a lot of hesitation to start with and comments such as, 'Oh, I can't think' or, 'I don't know what to say'. But if the helper perseveres and accepts any sort of response, however inappropriate at first, the mental reaction improves very quickly.

The helper asks the lipreader, 'What would you add to finish these sentences?'

Peter put on his coat and picked up his case and . . .
One wheel came off the lorry, then it swerved off the road and . . .
Before they booked for their holiday they made certain that . . .
As they turned the corner they saw . . .
As she ran out of the building she shouted . . .
I had just put down my shopping and sat down for a moment when . . .
While we were waiting for the plane to take off we . . .
Sometimes I think I am . . .

A similar exercise can be done by completing the lines of familiar songs. Of course if the lipreader says 'I don't know that' then go on to the next.

It's a long way to . . .
John Brown's body . . .
Drink to me only . . .
Should old acquaintance be forgot . . .
Rule Britannia . . .
I dream of Jeanie . . .
It's a great big shame . . .
Old MacDonald had a . . .

These may need changing to suit the generation gap.

Ten green bottles . . .
My bonnie lies over the ocean . . .

Or try well-known sayings used in everyday speech. The helper should read out the following and the lipreader complete each.

I'll do it this year, next year . . .
I told him, 'In for a penny . . .
We must stick together, it's 'All for one and . . .
He went about it with a hop, skip and . . .
They named their triplets Faith, Hope and . . .
If you have an early night it will make you healthy, wealthy and . . .
They were all there, every Tom, Dick and . . .
'It's all very well,' she said, 'but it's always jam yesterday, jam tomorrow but never . . .

It can also be done by asking for a number as an answer. How many?

Weeks in one year?
Pence in one pound?
Players in a football team?
Lives has a cat?
In a baker's dozen?
Princes in the Tower?
Men on a dead man's chest?
Commandments?
Tentacles on an octopus?
Teeth in an adult?
Rowing in a boat race crew?
Degrees in a right angle?
Dots in a semi-colon?

As mentioned earlier nursery rhymes again provide material that will be well-known. Even if the lipreader feels he has forgotten them, this is apparently untrue because it takes very little time to get into the way of remembering nursery rhymes.

Who pulled out a plum?
Who fell off a wall?
Who sang for his supper?
Who called for his pipe?
Who found a crooked sixpence?

Who had too many children?
Who found the cupboard was bare?
Who was under the haystack fast asleep?
Who shall have music wherever she goes?
Who met a pieman going to the fair?
Who licked the platter clean?

Characters from stories may also be sufficiently well-known to elicit a quick response:
Who was the boy who never grew up?
Who asked for more porridge?
Who wanted his pound of flesh?
Who thought Christmas was humbug?
Who rode to York on his horse Black Bess?
Who found herself on the other side of the looking-glass?
Who possessed a magic lamp?
Who shouted 'Off with his head!' once every minute!
Who married Lorna Doone?
Who slept for many years in the mountains of North America?
Who lived with his men in Sherwood Forest?
Who was shipwrecked and lived on a desert island?

There are other thought-inducing questions or statements. Tell me quickly three things which are found:
— in the sea
— in a museum
— in a toolshed
— in a toolbox
— in a jewel box
— in a left luggage department
— in a conservatory
— in a hothouse
— in a circus

Now can you tell me three:
— London mainline stations
— Shakespearian plays
— books of the New Testament
— bones of the body
— indoor games
— English members of Parliament
— of Henry VIII's wives

Any letter of the alphabet can be used to give a quiz similar to the following.

All the answers to this quiz begin with the sound ba (b). The lipreader should try to lipread the question and give an answer. It is not an intelligence test but an attempt to make you think as well as lipread.

This is an animal which, despite public belief, is colourblind. (Bull)

This weapon returns to the sender. (Boomerang)

This bush gives its name to a household tool. (Broom)

This insect was crushed to produce a purple dye for royal clothing. (Beetle)

This may mean a place to sit, or somewhere to leave your money, or something to rely on. (Bank)

This is one of the four tastes that the tongue can distinguish. (Bitter)

This is another name for a flag. (Banner)

In the song, we said goodbye to this bird. (Blackbird)

In Conclusion

These notes have been an attempt to give work that has been found useful in practice and which form a basis to encourage helper and lipreader to work together. In any skill, learning follows a pattern, being slow at the start, although there is often an initial uplift, with a good teacher, realizing that a standard is possible, then follow drill and the donkey work necessary for learning, with little evident progress. At this stage it is helpful for the lipreader to be taken back to an early exercise so that he can see how much easier it is for him to follow now. Then comes a 'hump' or sticking place where much encouragement is needed because little progress apparently takes place, until one day that appears to fade and more rapid progress is apparent.

Lipreading never stops, in that even the best at the skill find new language to attempt, new faces to present new problems, and practice is always necessary to maintain the standard reached. But, as with other skills, once accomplished it is an achievement for the lipreader to be proud of.

For the helper, it is necessary to maintain an expectant attitude, i.e. to expect the lipreader to feel depression when he cannot read something that appears simple, to expect discouragement when he appears not to know it all in a few weeks, to expect to have to cajole and repeat and repeat and repeat — all without showing signs of irritation or boredom. If either sets in then stop and wait until you both feel able to strike the right attitude again and do a little more. Your reward, if you seek it, is in the progress that your lipreader makes and that will be very dependent on your own approach to the practice sessions and your own enjoyment of them.

APPENDIX: WHAT THE SUFFERERS HAVE TO SAY

It is time the hard of hearing spoke for themselves. I have spoken from a life's profession, both working and living with the deaf, some of whom were born without sound, some dually handicapped, because an illness affecting the meninge of the brain is likely to cause a degree of hearing loss as well as a degree of brain damage; some rich and some poor in financial terms; some highly trained professionals, others working at humdrum tasks; some of high social standing, others not. In other words, deafness has been the great leveller and all have suffered alike. Because of these experiences it has been possible to gain a wide knowledge of how a loss affects people with different personalities in different jobs and from different backgrounds; but I thought that comments from the deaf themselves would enable anyone reading this book to identify utterly with the feelings and experiences they relate. The following paragraphs, therefore, have been sent to me from a wide range of past and present clients and I include them here unadulterated.

On lipreading:
'I am an elderly lady and very very deaf. You cannot learn to lipread in a fortnight as some people seem to think. You must get used to the others in the class who may be far worse than you as regards their hearing. To my mind, lipreading gives you a little or more (as the case may be) confidence to go among people. I thoroughly enjoyed every class I attended and learned quite a lot about deafness and hearing aids. Also I found it was an advantage to have a sense of humour and so to be able to laugh with others at my own mistakes.'

'As your hearing goes you will be lipreading automatically, as with a normal person in a very crowded, noisy place. So it will be a great help if you can go along to lipreading classes or join some club or organization for the hard of hearing. Having said that, lipreading is not the answer to all your problems; you will find you will have to use every bit of hearing you have left. When I see hearing people looking irritated this puts me off because it makes me feel ill at ease and then my lipreading goes to pot.'

'I find the uncertainty a great strain because one can only be as good a lipreader as the speaker is readable. It undermines one's confidence. We have to work so hard to keep up.'

'Within the confines of the classroom I do well but in the everyday world not so. Everything militates against the lipreader. The confusion of noise. People speak to the sky, to the pavement; their lips barely move or they whisper — and why not, if they can hear? They wear beards, as if moustaches weren't enough! They wave their hands in front of their faces and often obey the old Naval command 'Make smoke'. I ask you! But despite all this I am thankful that I decided to try and become a lipreader because, even with my aid, I cannot understand today the spoken word unless I can see the speaker, so where would I be without my lipreading?'

On social life:
'The best speakers are those who have passed the barrier of embarrassment, who know that it is possible to communicate with the deaf but they also know they have to make an effort too.'

'I find it so frustrating not being able to go to lectures. There are so many wonderful ones on paintings and furniture that I'd love to go to but it is useless.' (This from a professional interior decorator.)

'I rarely go out unless to tramp on my own. People cannot talk to you sideways on and very few like to walk along in silence.'

'The only social life I have is with the lipreaders in class. Sometimes a member of class will come and see me but we all live so far apart that this is not easy.'

'I've stopped going out to eat. While I eat I hear my own chewing sound echoing in my head so I have to stop listening while eating and I just miss things.'

'I'm so tired when I've concentrated at work that I'm thankful to sit indoors and not have to lipread anyone.'

'I do try to go out because I feel I shall lose all my friends if I don't make the effort but I find that, even when they have asked me, they leave me out of conversations or I probably laugh too loud and long at what I presume to be jokes because I often think they look at me strangely.'

Within the family:
'I always remember that it is not anyone else's fault that I am deaf, so I must make every effort to make it less trouble for them, otherwise why should they bother with me? After all, they naturally only see how difficult it is from their point of view and can't possibly be expected to realize what a struggle it is for the deaf.'

'By and large my wife has been very tolerant, especially as she is such a quick person herself. I left the activities pertaining to the boys' education to her. She had to see the Headmaster, go to school lectures, etc. It was all too easy for me to get things bottom upwards. But my inability to follow the cinema, theatre or anything of that sort has meant that she has made a social life for herself while mine has been work and home. I have always accepted this but always considered it tragic and deeply resented it. I am of the considered opinion that it is a very hard thing to be living with someone with a hearing loss. It must be very frustrating.'

'My wife gets very tired now because she has to be my ears. She has to answer the door, the telephone and contact workmen all the time, as well as remembering that I cannot understand her once we are out of sight. My boys have given up and I hardly ever manage a decent conversation with them now. Perhaps they think they are being kind in saving me the difficulty of lipreading but I do feel left out and no longer the mainstay of the family; I feel quite miserable about it really.'

'It took a long time for us to adjust and my wife still has to remember that I cannot hear. The trouble is I can lipread her so well that she forgets I need to be within eyeshot. We have made a different sort of life together because so many mutual friends stopped asking us out — perhaps they felt embarrassed. My deafness has brought us closer together but it has made as much difference to my wife as it has to me and I worry that she has to give up things.'

Other comments:
'I'm fortunate in being able to have the Visicom trial telephone facilities, funded by British Telecom. It has made a tremendous difference to my life. I always had to rely on getting someone to make calls for me — I still cannot have a truly private call but at least I can ring round for myself now.'

'The captions on television have altered my life. I don't feel so lonely and cut-off.'

'It was a great relief to me to lose the last particle of hearing, although I had started going deaf at twenty-one. It was a tremendous relief to my nerves. If one is deaf one has no alternative but to wear an aid but they are a distress to one's nervous system. I used to think of it as trying to read bad focus.'

I think a deaf person is probably a good driver. He is aware of hazards as he is looking for them more than the average driver and is probably concentrating harder.'

'I have come across one or two deaf people who seemed to be aggressive. The great tragedy is that it destroys confidence. It induces a kind of nervousness, a *too* great a desire to please, a tendency to laugh too soon. In the hearing world proper people are not like this. We are.'

'I always thought the deaf lived in a silent world. Now that I have become deaf I wish it was — the noises that plague me all the time are driving me mad.'

And from a hearing spouse:
'I never imagined that deafness could have such a shattering effect on us both. I felt helpless to do anything — still do, in fact. I do my best to write things down but find I keep so much to myself that we would formerly share. It's a very

sad, disturbing handicap and I never realised what an enormous part silly jokes and asides played in our lives.'

All the remarks above could have been repeated scores of times. The overall picture that comes through is one of initial disbelief that deafness is a debilitating handicap; then frustration that others do not truly understand the communication problems that arise; and often a final resignation that they never will and that life will be more restricted and less enjoyable from now on.

When asked what they thought would most help deaf people come to terms with their handicap and what would they like the public to do to help, all saw this as one and the same question and replied that the greatest relief would be to know that every member of the public would speak clearly and be made aware of the pitfalls of lipreading, so that communication could become a pleasure once more.

USEFUL INFORMATION

There are a number of splinter groups amongst services for the deaf, dealing with specific problems, for example, the Rubella Group who deal with the special problems of mothers who suffered German Measles during early pregnancy and whose children were born with a hearing loss.

The following societies and services are those more likely to prove useful to the deafened adult:

British Association for the Hard of Hearing
7/11 Armstrong Road
London W3 7JL
Tel: 01-743 1110/1353

General Membership is a very nominal sum and a directory listing the 220 clubs and area representatives is available free of charge.
The association produces a monthly magazine, arranges courses, meetings and holidays for the hard of hearing, as well as running social gatherings and lipreading classes.

Royal National Institute for the Deaf
105 Gower Street
London WC1E 6AH
Tel: 01-387 8033

The body covering all aspects of deafness. A journal is produced with a variety of news and information and includes the newsletter of the British Tinnitus Association.

These first two associations produce a large variety of leaflets covering such aspects as Special Aids to Hearing, The Deaf Person in Hospital, Lists of Hearing Aids and How to Install the Loop System, Clear Speech and Lipreading, Aids to Everyday Living, i.e. all aspects of the problem of communication.

The Health Council
78 New Oxford Street
London WC1A 1AH
Tel: 01-637 1881

Produces some useful pamphlets on how the public may help the hard of hearing.

The Association for Teachers of
   Lipreading to Adults
The Information Officer
c/o The Post Office
Slimbridge
Gloucester

A teaching body from which may be obtained details of your nearest lipreading class.

British Telecom produce telephone equipment and other signalling devices to help the handicapped.
   Your Telephone Sales Office will provide leaflets giving information on telephone couplers, watch receivers, special doorbells and lamps to help the deafened. Or the Yellow Pages section of the telephone directory will give you the number to contact for information on a wide range of services and apparatus.

British Deaf Association
38 Victoria Place
Carlisle CA1 1EX
Tel: 0228 20188

Concerned with both the born deaf and the deafened adult and produce useful leaflets. Their services include interpreters for the born deaf, social clubs, and social services for the blind/deaf and for deaf patients in hospitals.

Department of Health and Social Security
LASS/SH2C
Alexander Fleming House
Elephant and Castle
London SE1 6BY

Produce notes on general guidance for hearing aid users which are helpful for anyone issued with an aid, showing both how to wear it and use it to advantage.

Mention should be made of the *Sympathetic Hearing Scheme*, details of which may be obtained from the Royal National Institute for the Deaf.

The scheme uses a card showing the 'ear' symbol which has been approved as a sticker and an identity card for the use of deaf people. It aims at providing a basic training in communicating for any members of the public who work with deaf people and the card may be carried by all deaf persons to show when they require consideration at places displaying the symbol. The cards are plastic and available from the RNID.

The RNID also funds the *Hearing Dogs for the Deaf* scheme. Guide dogs for the blind have long been familiar but now it is possible for a deaf person to have a specially trained dog as a helper and companion.

The scheme was launched in 1982 but as each dog requires training and placement to the tune of several thousand pounds, funds are badly needed to ensure the future success of the scheme. Details of the scheme and its benefits are set out in a leaflet available from the RNID.

As well as devices provided through British Telecom, the RNID have many practical gadgets on sale. These include flashing light alarms, vibrator alarms, doorbells and entry phones, telephone amplifiers, Prestel and Viewphone, radio and television adaptors, fire and baby alarms — all of which may be seen at their offices or pamphlets sent for information and prices.

INDEX

pitch, 22
public attitude, 20, 28, 75, 81

recruitment, 40
rephrasing, 21
residual hearing, 29, 111

self-esteem, 67
sense of humour, 20, 26, 74, 80
sentence stress, 58
sound memory, 55
 volume of, 64, 168
 waves, 63, 64
speech, analysis, 93–97, 131, 145
 conversational, 66
 cued, 92
 discrimination, 47
 exercises, 142, 150–155
 faults, 136–137, 141

intensity level, 55–56
patterns, 23
perception, 56–57, 92, 109–110
teaching, 135, 148
volume of, 65
spondee words, 60

telephone amplifier, 28
television adaptor, 28
tinnitus, 16, 34, 36, 37
 association, 38–41, 78

vibration, 35, 138
voice, 133–134, 146
vowel discrimination, 47

Willis' parcusis, 108

Zund-Burguet, Dr, 42

In the same series ...

DEPRESSION
Its Causes and How to Overcome It

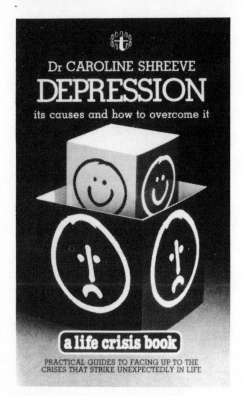

Dr Caroline Shreeve explains how depression — one of the worst imaginable wasters of human life and potential — can be conquered with simple self-help measures. An ex-sufferer herself, she talks with deep sympathy and understanding of the nature and symptoms of depression, and its psychological and biochemical causes. In an easy to follow three-stage plan she outlines how a personal programme of positive thought, combined with simple exercises and learning how to cope with stress, can put an end forever to this bewildering and devastating illness, and re-kindle your zest for life.